MAGIC OF
CATALYTIC HEALTH VITALIZERS

Also by the author:

*Extraordinary Healing Secrets from a Doctor's
Private Files*

*Doctor Van Fleet's Amazing New "Non-Glue-
Food" Diet*

MAGIC OF
CATALYTIC HEALTH VITALIZERS

James K. Van Fleet, D.C.

PARKER PUBLISHING COMPANY, INC.
WEST NYACK, NEW YORK

Library of Congress Cataloging in Publication Data

Van Fleet, James K
  Magic of catalytic health vitalizers.

  Includes index.
  1. Food, Natural—Therapeutic use. 2. Vitamin
therapy. 3. Diet therapy. I. Title.
RM237.55.V36   615'.854   79-22024
ISBN 0-13-545012-8

Printed in the United States of America

How Catalytic Health Vitalizers Can Improve Your Health and Increase Your Vigor

Many people suffer from chronic fatigue. They seem tired all the time. They have no pep—no energy or vitality. They drag from one task to another, not realizing that chronic fatigue is really not necessary at all. One of the common complaints I hear every day in my office, no matter what the major problem, is how the person feels so tired and worn-out all the time. In some instances, chronic fatigue is the primary symptom or the main complaint.

When I first began practice in 1949, I thought the lack of energy, or chronic fatigue, was a diseased condition all by itself, for I constantly heard comments like these from my patients: "Doc, I'm always so tired I feel as if I can't make it another day . . . I'm so worn-out all the time I can't even think straight . . . I just don't have any vitality whatever . . . I have no spark, no zip, no zest for living . . . I ache and hurt all over, I'm so tired . . . I drag around all day long . . . I wake up as tired as when I went to bed. . . ."

However, I soon discovered that chronic fatigue is almost

always the result of some other underlying condition, such as: anemia; low blood pressure; blood loss from bleeding ulcers or hemorrhoids; vitamin deficiency, especially of the B complex; malnutrition, particularly a lack of protein; some heart disorders; circulatory problems; chronic liver or kidney disease; colitis, diarrhea, constipation, and other troubles in the digestive tract; any focal infection, for example, the ear, sinus, and so on; an underactive thyroid gland; and many more conditions too numerous to mention.

I also found that getting rid of that tired, run-down, and worn-out feeling came about when the basic problem was corrected. Increased stamina and higher vitality were *fringe benefits* my patients enjoyed when their major illnesses were cured.

Now you might wonder at my use of the term, *catalytic health vitalizers. Catalysis* actually means the causing of a chemical reaction by the presence of a certain substance known as a *catalyst.* Although the catalyst must be present for the reaction to take place, its action is actually *secondary,* not primary.

The various catalytic health vitalizers I use in my practice are given to the patient *primarily* to cure the basic illness. But as a matter of course, the *secondary* reaction is to supply fresh stamina and energy to the patient.

So although the original or primary purpose of giving these substances to the patient is to correct his illness rather than restoring his energy (the secondary reaction), *the end result is always increased vitality, stamina and zest for living.* That is why I call them *catalytic health vitalizers.* They can include—but certainly are not limited to—natural foods, fruit and vegetable juices, vitamins, minerals, enzymes, herbs, and so on.

The benefits you'll gain for yourself from using these catalytic health vitalizers are tremendous. Not only will you be able to correct your major health problem, but you'll also gain the following benefits in energy, loss of fatigue, and overall well-being. I have seen these fantastic results demonstrated time and again in my practice. Let me tell you about some of them right now. Just for example:

INTRODUCTION

1. *You'll have more vitality, more energy and stamina, pep, and go-power.* You'll feel self-confident and be more sure of yourself. You'll no longer shun business or social activities because you don't feel up to par. You'll not have to make excuses that you're so run-down and worn-out you can't make it.

2. *You'll start looking ahead for new triumphs and new challenges.* You'll no longer live in the glories and successes of the past. You'll live in the ever-present now, today—not yesterday. Many of my older patients tell me they now have a new zest and zeal for life that was missing before they started using catalytic health vitalizers. As one of my patients said, "I now find life an experience to be enjoyed—not a problem to be solved."

3. *You'll feel at your peak and ready to tackle anything all the time,* not just part of the time, or now and then. Catalytic health vitalizers not only give you more immediate energy, but they also develop your endurance and staying power. If you feel your present health is satisfactory, I have good news for you. It will get much, much better.

4. *You'll be free from a grim collection of aches and pains.* When you hurt somewhere, you hurt all over. Your muscles tense and you burn up vital energy that is required for work that needs to be done. When you use catalytic health vitalizers, you'll find that as your aches and pains disappear energy returns. Where before there was weakness and fatigue, you'll now find strength and stamina. Not only that, but with your new reservoir of energy you'll find that ailments such as colds and the flu, as well as miscellaneous aches and pains, are not as troublesome, nor do they last as long as they used to.

5. *With catalytic health vitalizers, you'll no longer be nervous or high-strung.* You won't suffer with anxiety, depression, and irritability, all of which are a severe drain on your energy reserves. You'll have a brighter, more optimistic outlook on life. Your physical and mental performance will be greatly improved.

6. *Your sex life can improve dramatically.* No longer will you be too tired or use the excuse of a headache to avoid sexual relations with your partner. A vigorous continuing interest in sex

is a sign of good physical and mental health. I have patients in their seventies and eighties who have rediscovered a deep interest in sex after they thought they were all finished. And I might add that certain specific catalytic health vitalizers have given them the physical abilities to match their desires.

7. *You can look and feel at least 5 to 10 years younger*, if not more. After you start using one specific catalytic health vitalizer, you will find that your face no longer has a drawn, tense, and anxious appearance. As these lines of worry and fatigue disappear with the new energy that will be yours, you'll see a more youthful face appearing in the mirror each day. And you'll actually be able to lengthen your *prime of life.*

8. *You'll have increased energy and vitality* when you follow the guidance in this book. You'll also find that you'll be able to achieve new and higher health levels. Your resistance to disease will be much, much greater than before. You cannot possibly have vitality when you're tired and sick, and you can't help but have vitality when you're healthy and well.

To quickly summarize, then, let me say that if you want to have younger looking skin . . . better sleeping habits . . . shorter periods of sickness . . . less nervous tension . . . shinier hair . . . better teeth . . . a stronger heart . . . a calmer disposition . . . better eyesight . . . a more youthful appearance . . . an improved sexual vitality . . . better digestion . . . quicker reflexes . . . a smoother functioning metabolism, then use the catalytic health vitalizers I'll tell you about in this book. You'll be most happy that you did.

James K. Van Fleet, D.C.

Contents

CONTENTS

CONTENTS

CONTENTS

CONTENTS

11

CONTENTS

CONTENTS

CONTENTS

CONTENTS

CONTENTS

CONTENTS

1

How Catalytic Health Vitalizers Available Almost Anywhere Can Bring You New Vitality and Vigor

In my years of practice, I have found that many patients do not need prescription drugs or medicines to restore their good health or maintain their vitality. In fact, drugs so often cause such undesirable side effects that their use is highly questionable in many instances.

What to do then? Well, one way is to literally make your fruit and vegetable juicer your own drugstore. The benefits you can gain—with no undesirable side effects whatever—from the "natural medicines" found in this kind of catalytic health vitalizer—raw fruit and vegetable juices—are tremendous. For example:

CATALYTIC HEALTH VITALIZERS BRING YOU NEW VITALITY

1. Catalytic health energizers in the form of fruit juices act as cleansers of the body, especially the bloodstream, the kidneys and urinary system, and the digestive tract. They furnish the body with all the sugar it needs for energy in the form of natural carbohydrates. Fruit juices also supply the body with necessary minerals and vitamins, especially vitamin C.

2. Vegetable juices are the tissue builders and regenerators of the body. When properly extracted from fresh, raw vegetables having no chemical additives or preservatives, these catalytic health vitalizers contain most of the amino acids, minerals, enzymes, and many of the vitamins needed by the body.

3. People with bad teeth, dentures, or no teeth at all can get their nourishment from such catalytic health vitalizers as raw fruit and vegetable juices. Raw juices are also invaluable in helping a person recover from surgery or a prolonged illness. Invalids or elderly people who have lost their appetites can drink raw fruit and vegetable juices easily without having to force heavy, hard-to-digest foods into an unwilling digestive system.

4. Persons with ulcers normally cannot eat raw vegetables; yet they can readily drink raw carrot, celery, or cabbage juice and suffer no ill effects whatever. Juices are soothing, healing, and nourishing. They have no roughage to irritate the ulcerated areas.

5. Raw carrot juice is a magnificent kind of catalytic health vitalizer for babies. Milk can be mixed with it without curdling. It is excellent for growing children. It contains the minerals and many of the vitamins so necessary for growth and good health. Raw carrot juice also provides outstanding benefits to teen-agers. It helps in normal glandular development and minimizes the problem of adolescent acne.

6. Vegetable juices prevent constipation and gall bladder problems, both of which are closely related to the intake of soft, refined, man-made foods, and insufficient physical activity.

7. Such catalytic health vitalizers as fruit and vegetable juices, taken regularly, guarantee that your body is getting the proper amount of tissue-building materials. The energy they supply also insures you'll get a lot more enjoyment from your daily activities.

How Fred T's Health Was Amazingly Restored and His Energy Levels Built Up for Only Pennies a Day

Fred T. came to my office seeking help primarily for his digestive problem. He seemed unable to hold any solid food on his stomach. He had lost weight, was weak, and felt completely exhausted as a result of his inability to eat properly. A laboratory analysis of his blood revealed he was also suffering from anemia.

At the time Fred came to see me, I had become extremely interested in nutritional therapy as a helpful adjunct in my practice. After a complete study of Fred's case and his previous history, I decided upon raw carrot juice as the best catalytic health vitalizer for him.

In the beginning I asked Fred to drink a glass of carrot juice with each meal for a total of 3 a day. At the end of one month, we saw only a slight improvement, so we increased his intake to 2 quarts a day. We then saw a remarkable change for the better in both his health and strength. Fred was able to eat whatever he desired without any ill effect. He recovered completely from his anemia, gained 18 pounds, and is today the picture of robust health. He tells me his energy supply seems inexhaustible. He feels better than he has in years.

How This Catalytic Health Vitalizer Formed the Basis for a Surgical Diet

One of my patients, who was familiar with the benefits to be gained from raw carrot juice, used it to help her 60 year old husband recover from prostate surgery. Mildred said when Harry came home from the hospital he was still weak and exhausted. He had no appetite whatever. Mildred said he would just lie around, seeming despondent and acting as if he'd lost his will to live.

After a few days of watching Harry go slowly downhill, she decided to abandon the hospital diet and take matters into her own hands. She began giving Harry a quart of fresh raw carrot juice daily. His recovery was almost immediate. He regained his appetite, got his strength back, and was up and around, feeling quite normal again, in a week with the use of this marvelous catalytic health vitalizer.

How a Glaucoma Patient Regained Her Eyesight

My niece, Judy, is a county social worker who sees many people with health problems. Last year she met a 68 year old woman who had suffered with glaucoma for several years. This woman's eyesight had become so bad she was able to distinguish only between light and dark.

Then, on a neighbor's advice, she began eating 3 or 4 boiled carrots a day. She also drank the water the carrots had been boiled in. Slowly she began to gain back some of her lost eyesight.

My niece recommended to her that she drink raw carrot juice each day rather than eat cooked carrots, and her eyesight improved even more. Judy tells me this woman can now make out objects and identify certain colors, and although she cannot see who the persons are, she can tell when people pass by in front of her house or when they come up on the front porch.

Of course, this is not to imply that raw carrot juice alone can completely cure glaucoma; it cannot. But it does indicate how this specific catalytic health vitalizer can be of great benefit to the eyes and help healthy ones retain their vision.

Other Benefits You Can Gain from This Catalytic Health Vitalizer

Probably because of its sweet, delicious flavor, carrot juice is the most popular of all the vegetable juices. But it has much more than taste to make it worthwhile, for it contains almost all the vitamins and minerals needed by the body. It is especially high in vitamin A, which is known as the *healing vitamin*.

This makes carrot juice of great value in cases of sinus or nasal congestion, asthma, hay fever, bronchitis, and lung problems, or for infections or inflammations of any mucous membranes in the body, no matter where. Carrot juice, with its high vitamin A content, has been used successfully to improve the eyes, beautify the hair and skin, and restore one's pep, energy, and go-power. It is one of the most potent and powerful catalytic health vitalizers you can use to help you overcome fatigue, weakness, and drowsiness throughout the day.

A few years ago in my book, *Extraordinary Healing Secrets from a Doctor's Private Files,** I asked readers to write me in care of the publisher if they knew of some extraordinary or unusual treatment that had helped them in the past. The response to my request has been most gratifying. I have received hundreds of letters from people giving me their case histories in complete detail. The next 2 case histories are based on a couple of these letters.

How Homer F's Long-Standing Bladder Problem Was Cured Almost Overnight

"I read with great interest in your book, *Extraordinary Healing Secrets,* how cherries can help arthritis, rheumatism, and gout," Homer F. wrote. "I know they must be effective in these conditions for some of my friends suffering with arthritis have received tremendous relief and made a marked improvement from eating cherries. But that is not the reason I'm writing to you. I wanted to tell you how cherry juice helped another condition I used to have in the hope that someone else might find the information useful. . . ."

Homer went on to say he'd been having trouble for the past 7 years—actually since the age of 55—with not being able to hold his urine. He was getting up half a dozen times at night to go to the bathroom, which really disturbed his sleep.

In the daytime he was running to the bathroom every half hour or so. Whenever he went somewhere, he always looked around right away to find a restroom, for he knew he'd need to use

---

*James K. Van Fleet, *Extraordinary Healing Secrets from a Doctor's Private Files.* (West Nyack, New York, Parker Publishing Company, Inc.), 1977.

it before he left. As Homer put it, "My condition reminded me of the 80 year old man who said, 'I spend half my time looking for the bathroom and the other half using it!' Trouble was, I was a long way from being 80."

Homer had tried a lot of various remedies before he finally found the right one. He tried vinegar and honey, but that didn't help. Then he tried cranberry juice, but that didn't go any good either. He quit drinking coffee and regular tea and tried different kinds of herb teas, but he didn't get any better. His doctor gave him several different prescriptions, but none of them worked.

One day Homer went fishing with a friend, but he didn't catch any fish. He spent most of his time standing behind a tree. His friend, Bill, said to him, "Homer, I used to have the same problem you have. I couldn't hold my urine either. I got rid of my ailment by drinking black cherry juice. Why not try some? It sure can't hurt you, and it might do you a lot of good."

As Homer said in his letter, "Well, I thought, what the heck, I'd tried everything else, I might as well try Bill's remedy." He went to the health food store and got a bottle of black cherry juice concentrate. He says the results have been absolutely fantastic. In less than a week he stopped getting up at night. He sleeps straight through now from the time he goes to bed until it's time to get up. And in the daytime he doesn't have to run to the bathroom every time he turns around.

"I use one tablespoon of the black cherry concentrate in a glass of water with each meal," Homer says in conclusion. "That's all I do and my condition has been completely cured. I hope you can use my letter to help others get relief from bladder and urine problems. It's such a simple remedy it's hard to believe, but I know one thing for sure. It works!"

Cherry Juice Also Resolves Burning Urination Problem

Homer is not the only one who's been able to resolve a urinary ailment with black cherry juice. I received a letter from a lady who used black cherry juice for her rheumatism and found to her surprise and delight that it not only relieved her rheumatism, but it also cleared up a problem she'd had with burning urination.

In her letter she said that she'd spent a lot of money on doctors, trying to find a cure for her bladder problem, but none of them had ever helped her. Then she discovered black cherry juice. Now she can go to the bathroom and void normally without any burning or pain. "What a wonderful feeling of relief," she says.

How Cherries and Cherry Juice Can Help Your Kidneys and Bladder

Why do cherries and cherry juice help kidney and bladder conditons? Because they contain magnesium, iron, and a great amount of silicon, all of which act as an effective cleanser of the kidneys, the bladder, and the entire urinary tract. Black cherries contain more minerals than the light colored cherries and would, therefore, be preferable for kidney and bladder ailments. In my practice, however, I have found either one to be effective in the treatment of arthritis, rheumatism, and gout. Both of these catalytic health energizers are also highly effective in the restoration of a person's strength and elevation of his energy levels.

How This Catalytic Health Vitalizor Can Also Help Kidney and Bladder Problems

I personally have found cranberry juice to be one of the best catalytic health vitalizers a person can use to clear up kidney or bladder infections, even though Homer said in his letter that it had not helped him. Let me tell you briefly about 3 such cases.

1. Bert L., an 85 year old man, had a badly infected kidney. It was so bad that his urine was almost white with pus. Since he was a disabled veteran, he was entitled to care in the VA hospital. The doctors there used drugs and various medicines, and although his condition improved, it did not clear up completely. He was finally discharged with some renewable drug prescriptions and went home with instructions to come back in 30 days for a check-up.

Bert came to me to see if I could help. I asked him to drink a quart of cranberry juice every day to help acidify the urine and clear up the infection. He took no more drugs during this time. When he returned to the VA hospital a month later, the x-rays of his kidneys showed them to be in excellent condition. His urine was clean and clear.

2. One of my patients, Susie G., developed a bladder infection after a touch of the flu. I had her get some unsweetened cranberry juice from the health food store and drink as much as she could every hour or so. Within less than 24 hours she got marked relief. The infection was completely cleared up in only 3 days.

3. Another of my patients, Sally N., had a son who suffered from a chronic bladder inflammation. His ailment had not responded to antibiotics. Sally was told his condition was untreatable and he would just have to live with it. She brought Gene to me for help. I recommended unsweetened cranberry juice for him. His "incurable" condition cleared up almost immediately.

Cranberry juice comes close to being a specific catalytic health vitalizer for an infection or inflammation of the kidneys or the bladder because of its ability to acidify the urine and sterilize the entire urinary system. When treating these conditions, I always ask the patient to take from 3 to 5 thousand milligrams of vitamin C daily, for this will help clear up the condition even more rapidly.

Cranberry juice is also one of the best energy builders I know of. Of course, when a lingering infection is cleared up, the body's reserve energy levels rise immediately. I have also found that cranberry juice seems to make a person more alert and sharper mentally. In short, it is an excellent catalytic health vitalizer.

How Dorothy J. Got Rid of Her Stomach Ulcers Without Expensive Medicines or Painful Surgery

I know you'll gain a great deal of benefit from the following letter I received from a Mrs. Dorothy J. in response to my request for helpful remedies.

"I read with great eagerness your chapters on upper and lower digestive tract disorders in your book," Mrs. J. wrote. "I was curious to find out if you would say anything about a home remedy I have found to be extremely successful in curing stomach ulcers. When you did not, I decided to write to you.

"I had 2 stomach ulcers the doctor was treating me for. He had me on a bland diet of soft foods and had eliminated all spices, coffee, tea, and greasy or rough foods. I was also taking some antacid tablets to help control the pain.

"I wasn't making any progress, though. In fact, he x-rayed me again after 3 weeks of treatment and told me if things did not get better in another month or so, he would have to operate and take out a third of my stomach!

"Well, that I didn't want, so I decided to do some investigation on my own. My Aunt Martha, who lives on a small farm in the Ozarks hill country of northwestern Arkansas, is a great believer in folk medicine. She's nearly 90 and extremely active yet. I doubt if she's ever been to a doctor more than once or twice in her whole life. She says she doesn't trust them. So I wrote her and told her of my problem.

"She answered right away and said the cure was simple. 'Drink half a dozen glasses of raw cabbage juice every day for 2 or 3 weeks and you'll be well,' she said. 'Don't know why you wasted your money on a doctor, anyway. Why didn't you write to me in the first place?'

"Well, I figured I didn't have anything to lose except my ulcers, so I decided to try Aunt Martha's remedy. I bought a good vegetable juicer, got several heads of cabbage at the store, and set right to work. I started with 6 glasses of juice the first day like Aunt Martha said. I drank one at breakfast, mid-morning, noon, mid-afternoon, supper, and one before going to bed. Amazingly, by the end of the fourth day, to my surprise, I had no more pain!

"I kept this up for 3 weeks, 6 glasses of raw cabbage juice every day. Then I cut down to 3 glasses a day, one with each meal. I had gone off the bland diet the doctor had put me on and was eating anything I wanted to. My bowel movements were normal and regular. I felt terrific. In fact, I didn't want to go back to the doctor, but my husband insisted.

"When the doctor x-rayed me, to his surprise, he found no sign of an ulcer. He was flabbergasted for he couldn't understand what had happened. But I wasn't surprised at all, for all my symptoms had completely disappeared. I had absolutely no pain whatever. To tell the truth, I had become quite unaware of the fact that I even had a stomach for I had no discomfort at all.

"I still drink raw cabbage juice to keep my ulcers from coming back, but now I drink only one small glass every day with breakfast. It seems to act as a natural laxative for me for my bowels are much better than they were even before I had my ulcers.

"I thought you'd like to know about this remedy for it really works. Maybe it will help someone else avoid painful surgery and a doctor's expensive fees. Even if cabbage cost 5 dollars a head, it would still be cheaper and less painful than an operation."

Another Case of Surgery Prevented by Natural Methods

Shortly after I received Dorothy J's letter, I had the opportunity to test the healing capacities of raw cabbage juice. A businessman from Memphis, Tennessee, Sidney K., was on a trip throughout the southeastern states when he came down with an acute attack of severe abdominal pain.

The physician he went to told him he had a bad case of ulcers, and he recommended immediate surgery. Since this was not an emergency, the hospital would not admit him until his insurance company was informed and guaranteed payment. Because a weekend was involved, this took several days.

Although Sidney was not well enough to travel and return home, he was still ambulatory, so, dreading the surgery, he came to see me about his condition. I suggested that he drink 6 to 8 glasses of raw cabbage juice each day. He did so, and by the time his insurance company had guaranteed payment to the hospital, he felt well enough to return home, so he cancelled the operation.

Sidney wrote me not long ago to say he had continued to drink raw cabbage juice every day for 3 more weeks after he returned home. He then called his own doctor and made an appointment for a complete gastro-intestinal examination. Although some scar tissue from a healed ulcer could be seen in the x-rays, his own physician could find no sign of an active ulcer, and gave him a clean bill of health.

How You Can Cure an Ulcer at Home

If you have a peptic ulcer, you may find that it will respond almost miraculously to raw cabbage juice. The only drawback seems to be the formation of gas, because the juice has a powerful cleansing property. The gas comes from waste putrefactive matter in the intestines being broken down by the juice. This is only temporary. It will pass just as soon as the bowels are thoroughly cleaned out and free of toxic materials.

Admittedly, cabbage juice is not too tasty. But its flavor can be noticeably improved by the addition of carrot juice. In fact, cabbage juice mixed with carrot juice will not cause as much gas as cabbage juice alone, yet its therapeutic value is almost as great.

Cabbage juice is an excellent source of vitamin C, as well as A and B. It also contains an abundance of almost all the minerals, making it valuable for almost any condition of ill health. It is also one of the best catalytic health energizers you can use to build up your strength and energy, your vitality and vigor.

George K's Arthritis Miraculously Responds to Inexpensive and Painless Therapy

When George came to see me, he was almost completely helpless and in terrific pain from his arthritis. He had spent hundreds of dollars on prescription drugs, doctors, and a variety of "curative" methods. He'd tried eliminating certain kinds of foods, had short wave treatments, diathermy, massage, and so on, but nothing helped. He continued to get worse instead of better.

Three fingers on his right hand were completely immovable. He had bursitis in both shoulders. His back, from the neck down to the tailbone, caused him constant pain. His left leg and hip were so stiff that he walked with a pronounced limp. He had been taking aspirin in excessive amounts, which caused severe gastric bleeding and pain and had resulted in anemia.

I immediately placed George on 2 quarts of carrot juice and one quart of celery juice daily. In less than 3 months' time, all his pain was gone. Although his fingers were still stiff, they were no longer sore. Movement gradually returned until he gained full use of them again. His left hip and leg loosened up and he was able to walk without pain or a limp.

George had also been troubled with his prostate gland. He had to get up to go to the bathroom 6 or 7 times a night. He'd been going to a doctor once a week for massage and physical therapy, but with no improvement at all. This condition vanished completely at the end of 9 weeks.

Today, George has no sign whatever of arthritis, bursistis, neuritis, anemia, or prostate gland trouble. He has reduced his intake of carrot juice to one quart and celery juice to one pint daily. He tells me he feels completely alive and full of energy and vitality for the first time in many years. Although he is now 67, his physical appearance belies his age. He could easily pass for 55. What amazing benefits George has gained from these 2 fantastic catalytic health vitalizers.

**Other Benefits You Can Gain
from Celery Juice**

I have already discussed the benefits to be gained from the catalytic health vitalizer, carrot juice; so let me tell you now about celery juice.

It has a favorable soothing and calming effect on the nervous system and is one of nature's best tranquilizers, helping the person not only to survive the daily stresses and strains of today's busy world, but also to get a sound and restful night's sleep. This capability of celery juice to settle a person's nerves in itself acts to restore strength and energy levels. And, of course, with a good night's rest you'll have no more trouble with sleepiness at inappropriate times during the day.

Celery juice is also of great help in cases of arthritis and hardening of the arteries because of its peculiar power to dissolve unwanted calcium deposits.

Celery juice is high in its mineral content and contains sodium, magnesium, potassium, calcium, and sulphur. It is also an excellent source of vitamins A, B, and C. This abundance of vitamins and minerals makes it a potent and powerful catalytic health vitalizer.

What Apple Juice Can Do for You

Apple juice is a marvelous catalytic health vitalizer. It is one of the best energy builders you can use. The juice never tastes better than when it comes from fresh apples that are ground through a raw fruit and vegetable juicer. It is a good cleanser of the intestinal tract. Apple juice is mildly laxative and is of great assistance in clearing up minor cases of constipation, especially in children. This cleansing action does sometimes create minor problems of gas, but this is of little consequence, especially when the reason is understood.

Apple juice is also useful for the treatment of nasal or sinus congestions. It will help stir a sluggish pancreas back to normal activity. It also acts as a cleanser for the liver and gall-bladder. Since apple juice contains silicon, it is valuable for the hair, skin, and fingernails.

An Astounding Case History
As Told to Me by Nancy M.

I could not leave this chapter before telling you about my friend, Nancy M. A few years back, Nancy went to her doctor for a complete physical examination. She did not feel well at all. She was always tired and worn-out. She had lost weight and had a constant pain in the lower part of her back.

Her doctor discovered that her left kidney was functioning only at about 30 percent. However, surgery was not advised for Nancy at the time, for her doctor hoped for a recovery. But a check-up 6 months later showed that both kidneys were now affected and barely working. Her doctor said she had a rare disease known as pyo-nephrosis which would eventually destroy both kidneys. He gave her only one year to live.

Nancy was placed on a strict vegetarian diet. No meat whatever was allowed. But it did not help. She continued to lose weight and become weaker. Urologists and surgeons from several well-known clinics throughout the country were consulted, but they offered no hope whatever of recovery.

In the 10th month of her year to live, Nancy failed rapidly. She became completely bedfast and weighed less than 100 pounds. She began to pass bits of kidney tissue in her urine. Every specimen was loaded with blood and pus. She finally gave up hope completely and put all her earthly affairs in order. As she told me, she was prepared to meet her Maker.

One day a high school chum, Laura, came by to visit her. Nancy had not seen her in 20 years. Laura did not recognize her at all. She said, "Nancy, have you tried raw juice therapy yet?" Of course Nancy had not. She didn't even know what Laura was talking about.

The next day Laura brought her a book on the subject. Nancy read it avidly. Figuring she had nothing to lose, she decided to try the raw juice therapy, and began drinking a gallon—a gallon, mind you!—of fresh raw carrot juice daily, supplemented with a half gallon of a green drink consisting primarily of celery juice and cabbage juice. She ate no other food at all; she drank only these juices.

Five days after starting this regimen, Nancy began to breathe easier. She could feel a surge of new energy coming into her body. At the end of one week, she got out of her bed for the first time in 3 months and stood up. In 2 weeks Nancy was walking by herself around her bedroom without help. In a month she was getting around the entire house unassisted.

That was more than 3 years ago. It took a year for Nancy to regain her health and get her weight back up to normal. Her kidneys are now functioning properly and give her no trouble at all. You would never know that she had been sick or given a death sentence a few years ago. Nancy still drinks a quart of carrot juice daily and a quart of her green drink. She eats fresh fruit and vegetables. With the exception of eggs, she still avoids animal foods completely.

I would not blame you if you found it hard to believe Nancy's story. If I did not know Nancy myself and if I were not personally familiar with the details of her case, I'd be hard put to believe it. But I know for a fact her story is true.

How You Can Prepare These Health Restoring Catalytic Health Vitalizers in Your Own Home

The ordinary citrus fruit juicer is not capable of extracting the juices from such catalytic health energizers as cabbage, celery, carrots, and apples. The kind that must be used is a *fruit and vegetable juicer.*

Most health food stores have quality fruit and vegetable juicers in a variety of models and prices. Usually, the more chrome, the higher the price; the more plastic, the lower the price. The main requirement is utility, not beauty. Get a juicer that will separate the juice from the pulp and cellulose of the fruit or vegetable. That is really all you're interested in. *Prevention* magazine also carries advertisements for fruit and vegetable juicers. Sears Roebuck presently markets a relatively inexpensive model called an *Automatic Pulp Ejector and Juice Extractor.* I have never used this model; so I cannot vouch for its capabilities.

Although the vitamins, minerals, and enzymes in these catalytic health vitalizers are also available in highly concentrated forms, and I do recommend in certain cases that my patients take specific ones in a capsule or pill form, I have found that vegetable and fruit juices are always highly efficacious in curing many ailments as well as raising energy levels and furnishing my patients with new vigor and vitality.

Let me point out here that fruit and vegetable juices are not the only catalytic health energizers available to you. They represent only a few of the many I will tell you about in the chapters to follow.

2

Miracle Health Remedies That Can Restore Your Health and Vitality

Certain catalytic health vitalizers are so efficient in their healing functions in the body that they truly deserve to be called "Miracle Health Remedies." Yet none of them are expensive to buy or hard to obtain. They can be found at your local supermarket or health food store. And the wonderful part about them is that not only will they solve a specific health problem for you, but they will also act as fantastic body energizers that help you get rid of fatigue, weakness, and that tired washed-out feeling—restoring your vigor, vitality, and zest for living.

35

Stubborn Prostate Problems Cleared Up
Quickly and Easily: Several Case Histories

One of the most troublesome problems for men over the age of 60 is an enlarged prostate gland. The enlarged prostate projects into the bladder and impedes the normal passage of urine. Typical symptoms include a constant desire to urinate, decreased size and force of the urinary stream, terminal dribbling, getting up several times a night to go to the bathroom. In extremely severe cases, prolonged urinary retention can result in progressive kidney failure and uremic poisoning.

Some men try to accept an enlarged and painful prostate as an inevitable consequence of old age; others turn to surgery for an answer to their problems. However, in a great many cases, neither of these two courses of action is necessary. Often the problem can be resolved quickly and easily. Let me give you several examples:

1. WILL B. GAINS AMAZING RESULTS
IN CHRONIC PROSTATE AILMENT

Will B. was suffering from a severely swollen and painful prostate gland when he came to see me. It was extremely difficult for him to urinate, and as he told me, it seemed to take forever and a day to get the stream started.

There was also a decrease in the force of the urinary stream; it was much smaller in diameter than before. As a result, Will's bladder was not being completely emptied, so he found himself trying to urinate every 20 minutes or so. But he could void only a small amount each time, usually dribbling just a few drops. Will was getting up a dozen times a night to go to the bathroom. He was suffering from a severe pressure pain in the lower abdomen over the bladder. This was especially noticeable upon palpation during his physical exam. He had a continual dull ache across the small of his back.

Will had been to a urologist before coming to my office. This doctor had recommended surgical removal of the prostate. That is actually why Will came to see me. Since the urologist had told

Will the prostatic enlargement was not cancerous, he wanted to try something else first that was not as drastic as surgery.

Will was exhausted from lack of sleep. He was nervous and extremely despondent about his condition. He'd lost several pounds and was thin, pale, and haggard when I first saw him. Physical examination of his prostate revealed that it was badly swollen and inflamed. It was extremely painful and tender during palpation.

Since I'd had marked success in treating benign enlargements of the prostate gland with bee pollen tablets, I recommended the same procedure to Will. I had him take 8 tablets daily, 2 with each meal and 2 just before going to bed. In less than 30 days, his severe symptoms had decreased considerably. At the end of 2 months, they had disappeared completely.

Will's urologist examined him again 3 months after he came to me. He told Will that although he still had some enlargement, it was now not enough to warrant surgery, especially since the previous inflammation causing his symptoms had "mysteriously" subsided.

Will has continued to have a check-up every 6 months by his urologist. This is an extremely wise precaution since cancer of the prostate is one of the commonest forms of cancer in older men. Although a year and a half has now gone by, no further action has been necessary. To play it safe, however, Will still takes 8 bee pollen tablets every day.

Will no longer becomes fatigued easily. In fact, he walks a couple of miles every day. He seems full of boundless energy and zest for living, even though he is now 73 years old. Will is in superior health, a far cry from when he first came to see me. For his condition, bee pollen was the perfect catalytic health vitalizer. It worked like magic to solve his problem.

2. HOW LLOYD R'S SEVERE PROSTATE PROBLEM WAS QUICKLY SOLVED

Continual progress is always being made by a relatively few far-sighted doctors in using such items as fruit and vegetable juices, natural foods, vitamins, minerals, herbs, and the like to treat disease naturally. Although I am not a scientist engaged in research as such, I have continued to look for new methods and new ways of combatting disease and helping my patients. The use of the catalytic health energizer, zinc, to heal Lloyd R's enlarged prostate is an example of this.

A few years ago, Lloyd, who was then 65, began to suffer with all the symptoms of an enlarged and inflamed prostate gland. At that time, Lloyd was advised by his doctor to resort to surgery to correct his condition, but he was not yet ready for such a drastic procedure. Instead, he came to my office to see if I could help him resolve his problem and avoid an operation.

Lloyd was exhausted. He was listless and had no energy whatever. His face was haggard and lined from lack of rest. My physical exam revealed a badly swollen and painful prostate gland. A complete dietary analysis showed that Lloyd was deficient in zinc.

This finding confirmed some recent health literature I had been reading about the deficiency of zinc in infections and inflammations of the genito-urinary tract, so I decided to use it along with bee pollen tablets to treat Lloyd's condition.

I had Lloyd take 30 milligrams of zinc daily, 10 milligrams with each meal along with 8 bee pollen tablets, 2 with each meal and 2 before going to bed. Lloyd responded quite rapidly. In less than 10 days, his condition improved markedly. It continued to do so, and at the end of only 30 days he had no sign of a prostate problem. He could urinate without any discomfort whatever. He slept all night without getting up unless he drank too much liquid before going to bed. Even then he had to get up only once, and his urination was completely normal again.

With undisturbed rest, Lloyd quickly recovered his lost energy. He no longer had that tired, drawn, and worn-out look on his face. He once again felt that life was well worth while. Truly, zinc is a marvelous health energizer to help restore health, energy, and strength to a sick person, no matter what the condition is.

Today, I routinely use both bee pollen tablets and zinc to heal inflamed and swollen prostate conditions. I have found that although bee pollen alone will resolve a prostate problem, zinc speeds up the healing process tremendously, so that a person's discomfort is relieved much more quickly.

I have also learned of several other methods of treating prostate problems from some of my patients. The following case history is one such example:

3. IRVIN E. USES EXTRAORDINARY AND DIFFERENT METHOD TO GAIN RELIEF

Irvin E., a patient of mine, told me that a few years ago a very painful prostate condition was causing him to go to the bathroom several times a night. His problem was so severe he was considering immediate surgery until he happened to read in a health magazine about a doctor using pumpkin seeds successfully for prostate problems. Irvin began eating pumpkin seeds, literally by the handful, and, amazingly, he found his condition vanished in only a few weeks. Although Irvin was coming to me for a different health problem, I examined his prostate gland after he told me this and found it to be completely normal.

Shortly afterward, I had a prostate problem case that did not respond completely to my zinc and bee pollen therapy. Although he was much improved, Elbert J's symptoms had not totally disappeared, so I decided to use Irvin's method with some minor changes.

Since pumpkin seeds are so rich in unsaturated fatty acids, I decided to use unsaturated fatty acid capsules. Elbert was 79 years old and wore false teeth, so pumpkin seeds were almost impossible for him to chew, but he had no trouble at all swallowing the capsules.

I had him take 4 a day, one with each meal and one before bedtime. His condition responded immediately to this treatment and his remaining symptoms soon disappeared. I feel this additional therapy must have been necessary because of Elbert's age and the length of time the condition had existed.

Benefits That You, Too, Can Gain from This Therapy

I have used a good portion of this chapter to discuss prostate problems and their solution, for I know how troublesome they can be to so many men over the age of 60. If you are having a prostate problem yourself and your doctor says your condition is not cancerous, then the bee pollen, zinc, and unsaturated fatty acid therapy would certainly be preferable to surgery. If you take 8 bee pollen tablets daily (2 with each meal and 2 before going to bed), 30 milligrams of zinc (10 with each meal), and 4 unsaturated fatty acid capsules (one with each meal and one before going to bed), you could easily find your problem solved or greatly minimized within 30 to 90 days.

Even if you're under 60 and not yet troubled with a prostate condition, you would be wise to use this same procedure as a precautionary measure so you could avoid the problem completely when you do get older. You could save yourself years of untold pain and misery with these 3 catalytic health vitalizers.

A great many other health problems can also be resolved by the use of bee pollen, zinc, and unsaturated fatty acids. I will discuss some of these in later chapters.

Peggy V. Gets Amazing Relief for Obstinate Skin Rash from Her Kitchen Cupboard

As I mentioned just a few moments ago, I have always been on the lookout for new methods and innovative procedures in combatting disease. However, in some instances, I've had to turn backward in time to find the right answer. Let me give you one example of this:

Peggy V. came to see if I could help her get rid of a rash on her left hand which she'd had for 3 years. It had started with her ring finger and spread until it covered almost all the back of her hand It caused her a great deal of discomfort, for it itched constantly. The appearance also caused her to feel embarrassed and she wore gloves most of the time when she went out of the house.

She had tried many things to clear it up—petroleum jelly, vitamin A ointment, vitamin E oil, rubber gloves, and so on—but nothing seemed to help. A dermatologist diagnosed her condition as a kind of eczema, but his prescription for some salve only made it worse.

Since Peggy had already tried several remedies which are often helpful in clearning up skin problems—especially vitamins A and E—I knew I had a real problem case on my hands. So I turned to my "kitchen remedy" reference file. There I found an old household remedy my own grandmother had given me for skin rashes and eczema: 2 teaspoons of blackstrap molasses taken internally twice a day, morning and night.

Peggy was reluctant to use this treatment, for it seemed too simple to her after 3 years of misery and dozens of more sophisticated remedies that had failed, but she finally agreed to try it for at least 30 days. At the end of 2 weeks she found her hand was almost clear. She could bend her fingers without pain or without cracking the skin on the back of her hand for the first time in years. The itching had stopped completely. The skin remained quite red for nearly 60 days, but at the end of that time, the color became normal again.

To Peggy, after 3 years of continual pain, itching, cracked skin, misery, and embarrassment, the cure seemed almost like a miracle. She continues to take the blackstrap molasses every day, for as she says, it's cheap medicine, and she doesn't want to run the risk of a relapse.

Not only that, but Peggy has found that her energy levels have gone up with her use of the molasses. She has more vigor and vitality, and since she has not changed any of her eating habits, her increased energy can only be credited to the blackstrap molasses.

Benefits You Yourself Can Gain
from This Catalytic Health Vitalizer

You do not have to have a skin rash or eczema to enjoy the marked benefits of blackstrap molasses. If you want to get rid of that run-down and worn-out tired feeling, blackstrap molasses could easily be the answer to your energy problem.

Blackstrap molasses has often been made fun of by some people who say it is a *fad food* eaten only by *health nuts*. Let me tell you a little bit about how it is made so you can understand why it is *not* just a fad food.

Both sugar and molasses come from the sap of the sugar cane. The sap is boiled, and the first extraction from it is crystallized raw sugar. The second extraction produces a light molasses, richer in vitamins and minerals than the raw sugar. But the third extraction, which produces the blackstrap molasses, is the richest of all.

Chemical analysis shows that blackstrap molasses contains the following vitamins and minerals: Inositol, thiamin (B-1), riboflavin (B-2), niacin (B-3), pyridoxine (B-6), pantothenic acid, biotin, calcium, phosphorus, iron, copper, and potassium.

Some nutritionists say blackstrap molasses has been found to recolor hair. It has also been credited with stopping falling hair. Because of its high iron content, it can prevent or help cure anemia.

When it comes to increasing energy levels, blackstrap molasses is much more economical and efficient to use than a certain well-known, over-the-counter product that uses iron, the vitamin B complex, and alcohol. Blackstrap molasses is an excellent catalytic health energizer well worth using no matter what the health problem might be.

Frank G's Shingles Healed in Two Weeks
with Spectacular Results

Frank came to me with an exceptionally bad case of shingles. Before the actual eruption he had suffered with chills and fever, he felt worn-out and run-down, and his stomach was upset, causing him to have a severe case of diarrhea. After 5 days of this, the typical shingles eruption appeared on his back and spread around his ribs and waist. The painful itching in the area of the lesions was extremely severe.

Having had a great deal of success in treating shingles with vitamin E, I recommended this procedure to Frank. I had him use a perle of vitamin E (containing 400 international units) on the infected area 3 times a day, morning, noon, and night. His wife simply pricked a pinhole in the vitamin E capsules and then rubbed the oil on the lesions. I also asked Frank to take 3 capsules of vitamin E daily.

Within 2 weeks, both the pain and the rash had disappeared. Frank's wife was greatly surprised. She is a registered nurse and was used to seeing shingles drag on for month after month. Needless to say, Frank was extremely pleased with the results.

Even after his shingles were healed, Frank continued to take 1,200 units of vitamin E daily—3 capsules of 400 international units, one with each meal—for he said they gave him a definite energy lift. This is not at all surprising, in view of how vitamin E functions physiologically in the body.

For instance, vitamin E helps conserve oxygen and helps the body tissues use oxygen more efficiently. Unless there is sufficient oxygen in the bloodstream to replace the carbon dioxide that results from physical or mental activity, a person will feel tired and worn-out, sluggish and sleepy. Vitamin E helps the process of exchanging oxygen for carbon dioxide.

How This Catalytic Health Vitalizer Can Help You, Too

Vitamin E can be especially important to you if you live in a smog area such as New York, Los Angeles, or any other large metropolis. Two of the main air pollutants in a highly industrialized area are ozone and nitrogen oxide, both of which are damaging to lung tissue. In animal laboratory experiments, it has been found that vitamin E given in therapeutic doses will protect the lungs from these agents.

Doctor Daniel B. Menzel, formerly of the Battelle Institute, and Director of pharmacology and medicine at Duke University in Durham, North Carolina, applied the knowledge gained in these animal experiments to humans. He found it took at least 200 international units of vitamin E daily to reverse the damage to human lungs from air pollutants.

Dr. Wilfrid E. Shute, a Canadian medical doctor, is a pioneer in the discovery and use of vitamin E in a variety of diseased conditions. He says that people living in today's environment are subjected to so many different toxic substances in the air and water, and so many chemicals in food, that virtually everyone needs to take, as a minimum, 200 to 800 international units of vitamin E daily to counteract these toxic substances.

Without a doubt, vitamin E, then, is a marvelous catalytic health vitalizer. It helps the body eliminate toxins, including carbon dioxide, and increases oxygen utilization. As the efficiency of oxygen use increases, so do energy, vigor, and vitality levels. Vitamin E is also a specific catalytic health vitalizer for cardiovascular conditions. I'll discuss that function of it in a later chapter along with many of its other outstanding benefits.

Sarah H. Uses a Different Method to Get Rid of Shingles and Gain Wonderful Relief

Sarah told me about a method she used to treat a case of shingles at home, with fabulous results. When she first broke out with the shingles, Sarah went to a dermatologist. Her symptoms were quite typical of a shingles case: fever, chills, malaise, breaking out on the back in the thoracic region, and on around the rib cage to the abdominal area. She had a great deal of burning pain and itching along the path of the eruption.

After several days of using the lotion the dermatologist had prescribed, it became apparent to Sarah that her condition was not improving; so she consulted some library books on home medical treatment. After analyzing and considering several remedies, she settled on the herb, golden seal.

She dissolved golden seal powder in boiled water and used

that to saturate the broken-out area of her skin several times a day and before going to bed at night. To speed up the healing process, she also took golden seal root powder internally—one capsule before each meal. Sarah said the eruption started drying up immediately, and in only 2 weeks she was completely healed and free of the shingles.

What Golden Seal Can Do for You

Golden seal can be used for many more ailments than shingles. It is one of the most wonderful remedies in the entire herb kingdom. When one considers all that can be accomplished by its use, and what it can actually do for a person, it almost seems like a real cure-all, a true miracle medicine food.

Golden seal is, according to many authorities, a most excellent natural remedy for colds, the flu, and all sorts of stomach and liver troubles. For open sores, inflammations, infections, eczema, ringworm, erysipelas, or any skin disease, golden seal is superior. That is why it was so successful in curing Sarah's shingles.

Golden seal is useful in inflammations of the mucous membranes and is extremely helpful in cases of intestinal troubles, such as colitis or diarrhea. It aids digestion and improves the appetite, thus increasing one's feeling of good health, vigor, and vitality.

I do want to mention that golden seal is an especially potent herb. Health practitioners with a great deal of experience and expertise in its use say that probably no more than one-third of a teaspoon should be taken internally in one day. Golden seal root powder can be obtained at any good health food store.

Ella V's Bladder Ailment Cured with Startlingly Different Procedure

Ella had suffered periodically with a recurring bladder infection for a dozen years and more. Her family physician had used many drugs, including the sulfas and various antibiotics, such as penicillin and aureomycin, for her condition, but even though these gave her some temporary relief, they never obtained permanent results, for in only a few weeks or a month or so, her infection would always return. Ella was bothered by these sieges from 4 to 6 times every year.

After her husband, Greg, had been successfully treated in my office for a different condition, Ella decided to try the drugless method of healing; so she came to see me. After going over my reference file of natural health remedies, I decided to have Ella try watermelon seed tea for her condition. I did not want to use anything stronger that might irritate her inflamed bladder even further, and I knew that the mild watermelon seed tea would not bother her.

I had Ella drink a cup of the tea 4 times a day: breakfast, dinner, supper, and early in the evening. How successful has this treatment been for her? Well, you can judge for yourself. Ella has now gone 18 months without any sign of a bladder infection. She says she has never felt better in all her life. Now that this nagging chronic infection has been relieved, her energy levels have gone up and she no longer feels depressed, despondent, and miserable about her life. To say it quite simply, Ella is one happy woman.

How This Treatment Could Help You

If you have been troubled with a recurrent bladder infection that causes burning or cloudy urine, as so many women are, then watermelon seed tea could be just the thing for you.

It is ever so simple to make. Crush two teaspoons of the dried seeds and steep them in a cup of hot water for an hour. Stir and strain. Drink a cup of this tea four times a day. To improve the flavor, you can add one of the natural teas, such as spearmint.

How do watermelon seeds work? They contain an ingredient known as *cucurbocitrin* which dilates the capillaries and reduces the pressure upon the larger blood vessels in the body. Watermelon seeds also act as a diuretic. This makes the tea made from them valuable in mild cases of high blood pressure where the doctor has prescribed a water pill such as hydrochlorothiazide (also known as oretic, esedrix, and hydrodiuril).

I should also point out here that inflammation of the bladder and burning urine occur most often in people who have excess acid in their systems caused by a high consumption of man-made sugars and starches. A diet high in fruits and low in man-made foods is extremely helpful in such cases. Fruits are especially valuable, for they are rich in alkaline salts and help to overcome the excess uric acid that is present.

How Sam N's Kidney Stones Were Dissolved with Extraordinary Treatment

I know of nothing that will sap a person's energy and strength more quickly than pain. I also know that the passage of a kidney stone is one of the most excruciating pains a person can have. It will cause a strong man to scream in agony. As one woman told me, "The pain of a kidney stone passing is the closest thing to having a baby that I know of."

Sam N. was especially familiar with this horrible pain. For the past four years he had been getting a kidney stone attack every two or three months. When this happened, he would have to be rushed to the hospital and get a shot of Demerol to ease the pain and pass the stone. After a few hours, he would be able to function again.

But he always lived in fear of not being able to get to the hospital during an attack, for the pain was almost unbearable without some sort of drug. So Sam came to me to see if I could help.

My dietary analysis revealed that he was grossly deficient in calcium, magnesium, and pyridoxine (vitamin B-6). Sam told me he had tried to restrict his calcium intake, hoping to prevent any further kidney stone formation, but he had not been successful. In fact, he had only compounded a bad situation, for now he had other problems directly traceable to the calcium shortage, specifically: nervous exhaustion and a cardiac irregularity. His heart was palpitating occasionally and skipping beats.

I asked Sam to take 150 milligrams of pyridoxine each day. I also had him take a high potency vitamin B supplement 3 times a day so he would have a balanced vitamin B intake with the pyridoxine. I gave him magnesium tablets as well as dolomite for his calcium and magnesium shortage. Here's why those supplements were needed:

Kidney stones are primarily formed of calcium oxalate. Magnesium helps hold the oxalic acid in solution in the urine, preventing it from precipitating out as oxalate particles that can eventually clump together with calcium to form kidney stones.

Vitamin B-6 helps control the body's production of oxalic acid, thus limiting the amount that reaches the kidneys. I also asked Sam to avoid foods that are high in oxalic acid, such as chocolate, cocoa, tea, rhubarb, spinach, chard, parsley, and beet tops.

Even though kidney stones are most often composed of calcium oxalate, I had Sam take dolomite, which contains both calcium and magnesium, and I had him eat plenty of calcium-rich foods since his body was so starved for calcium. As long as he got the magnesium and pyridoxine he needed to keep minerals in solution in the urine, the amount of calcium in his diet would not be a contributing factor in the formation of kidney stones. A person simply cannot go without calcium and remain in good health. Calcium is an absolute must, especially in cases of nervous exhaustion and cardiac irregularities.

What have been the results? Sam has been my patient now for nearly 2 years. He has never been back to the hospital once during that time for the passage of a kidney stone. His nervous exhaustion vanished within a month after he came to see me. His heart beat is now strong and regular with no sign of a skipped beat or any other irregularity. Sam now leads a happy, healthy, normal, and active life. He has more pep and energy than most people in their 30's and 40's, and Sam is now approaching 70.

How You Can Use These Catalytic Health Vitalizers Yourself

Although 3 catalytic health vitalizers were used to restore Sam's health—pyridoxine, calcium, and magnesium—let me discuss only 2 of them, calcium and magnesium. I will take up the benefits of pyridoxine later when I talk about the entire B complex.

Most people think of calcium only as a bone builder. It has many other functions. It is necessary for proper blood clotting, muscular activity, and the functioning of the nervous system.

Calcium has powers as a nerve tranquilizer to overcome irritability and grouchiness, as a calming and sedative agent to help insomniacs sleep better, and as a pain killer. As Doctor Harold Rosenberg, past president of the American Society of Preventive Medicine and a nutritional authority, says, "A calcium overdose is impossible."

Magnesium is related to calcium. It is necessary for the bones, teeth, and soft tissues. Too much sugar in the diet can lower magnesium absorption. Excessive use of alcohol can deplete magnesium stores. People who use diuretics, such as hydrochlorothiazide for high blood pressure, lose magnesium along with the water. Professor Roger Williams, author and biochemist, says a mild magnesium deficiency may be widespread and a disastrous deficiency may not be uncommon among those suffering from heart attacks.

The National Academy of Science's Food and Nutrition Board says that animals fed moderately low levels of magnesium, *sufficient to allow normal growth and prevent all gross signs of deficiency*, often develop calcified lesions of the soft tissues and increased susceptibility to the atherogenic effects of cholesterol feeding. In short, a subclinical magnesium deficiency can lead to harmful mineral deposits in the soft tissues, and no doubt, to kidney stones as well.

The best source of both calcium and magnesium is dolomite. This is a naturally occurring inexpensive substance that contains calcium and magnesium in their natural proportions, approximately 2 to 1. Enough dolomite should be taken to get at least 1,000 to 2,000 milligrams of calcium daily. The proper amount of magnesium will then accompany the calcium. There is no possibility whatever of any danger from an excess of dolomite. It is safe in any conceivable supplement quantity.

3

How These Special Invigorating Foods Can Act As Terrific Health Vitalizers Within Your Body

Over the years, I have compiled a list of a few special invigorating foods that could almost be called wonder *foods*. These foods are not panaceas; they will not cure everything, but they are terrific catalytic health vitalizers. They deliver more pep, energy, and go-power than the average food. They also give you a tremendous energy reserve. These special foods can heal a great many ailments, as you will soon see.

I would like to mention that it is impossible for me to include in this book all the case histories I have on file in my office. I have chosen only a few that are representative of the whole.

How Margaret L's General Health Was Incredibly Improved with This Special Catalytic Health Vitalizer

One of the readers of a previous health book of mine, Margaret L., wrote to give me the following story of her amazing recovery with this special catalytic health vitalizer.

Margaret had been bedridden for a number of years with a heart condition. She was troubled with an abnormally high cholesterol level and excessive hypertension. Her doctors had literally given up hope of any possibility of improvement. They had tried a variety of cholesterol-lowering medications, but none of them had been even remotely successful.

Then one day a friend, who had whipped her own high cholesterol problem with lecithin, suggested to Margaret that she try lecithin herself "just to see what might happen." Although Margaret had no hope of any change in her condition, she agreed to try her friend's recommendation. She used both lecithin granules and lecithin capsules. She sprinkled lecithin granules on her salads and also used lecithin in fruit juices, soups, and gravy. She used 6 to 8 tablespoons of granules each day. Margaret also took three 1,200 milligram lecithin capsules daily, one with each meal.

To her great surprise, Margaret's health began to improve almost immediately. Her doctors were amazed at the changes that took place. At the end of only 2 months, Margaret got out of bed and stayed out. Her cholesterol level dropped to normal in only 3 months, due only to the addition of lecithin to her food intake, for no other changes were made in her diet. At the end of 5 months, her high blood pressure dropped and returned almost to normal with readings of 130 to 135 over 85 to 90.

At the end of 6 months, Margaret felt better than she had in years. She was no longer bothered by dizzy spells or the headaches that had plagued her so badly before. In fact, Margaret said she did not suffer any more aches or pains anywhere in her body. Her energy levels rose dramatically, and she began doing tasks around the house that she had not done for months and years before.

How This Potent Catalytic
Health Vitalizer Can Help You

Lecithin is an absolutely amazing "wonder food." It can help you in any number of ways. For instance, many of my female patients have been most happy to find out that lecithin helps to distribute body weight more evenly. It takes it off where they don't want it and puts it on where they do.

Cases of heart troubles—as in Margaret's case—as well as angina pectoris, myasthenia gravis, and high cholesterol levels, have all responded favorably to lecithin. Some nutritionists feel it may aid in preventing the formation of gallstones.

I personally have found lecithin to be especially efficient in helping to lower blood cholesterol. Under certain circumstances, excessive cholesterol in the blood stream can become deposited in the blood vessel walls and cause hardening of the arteries, elevated blood pressures, and possible stroke.

Now most doctors try to prevent high blood cholesterol by reducing the amount of cholesterol in the diet. Eggs, for example, have been condemned by many physicians because of the high cholesterol content of the yolks. Yet an egg is one of nature's most perfect and complete foods, for it is rich in vitamins, minerals, and essential amino acids. Butter has also been blamed for high cholesterol levels in the bloodstream, but the tide of medical opinion is slowly changing on this point. Most experts in nutrition now agree that because butter is a natural food, and since it is completely liquid at body temperature, it should not be avoided.

So diet alone is not the direct answer to a high cholesterol problem. You see, cholesterol is made right within our bodies, and this internally manufactured cholesterol can be deposited in the arterial walls, *even of a person who consumes absolutely no cholesterol at all.*

Not only that, but the rate of cholesterol production in the body is inversely related to the amount of cholesterol coming in

53

from the outside. In short, not eating enough cholesterol-rich foods, such as eggs and butter, can open the body's cholesterol control valve, and speed up the production of cholesterol within the body.

The important point to keep in mind is not how much cholesterol is in the bloodstream, but how much is actually being deposited in the arterial walls. Now here is where your intake of lecithin becomes so important. Lecithin is an emulsifying agent, causing fats to either go into solution or remain in solution; so its presence in the bloodstream keeps cholesterol from precipitating out to be deposited in the arterial walls. It also helps dissolve the cholesterol that has already been deposited.

Doctor Lester M. Morrison, M.D., found that nigh blood cholesterol levels in patients were lowered when they consumed one ounce of lecithin daily for 3 months. Doctor Roger Williams, Ph.D., the famous biochemist and author of numerous books on nutrition, says that a better answer to the problem of cholesterol deposits is not to avoid cholesterol, but to consume more lecithin in the diet.

Summing up, then, lecithin is a natural food that can help your cardiovascular system. It can increase your vigor, vitality, pep, and go-power. It is an excellent catalytic health vitalizer to raise your energy levels.

How This "Miracle Food" Remarkably Acts As a *Lasting* Energy Pick-Up

Lack of energy is one of the constant and most common complaints I hear in my office every day of the week, not only from older persons, but also from young people as well. Of course, a variety of ailments such as hypoglycemia, anemia, low blood pressure, and chronic infections as well as vitamin, mineral, and other dietary deficiencies can also cause chronic fatigue and excessive weariness. However, I have found that even when these various problems are corrected the lack of energy is often still present. Brewer's yeast is the best solution I know of for this lack of energy problem.

I have also had scores of patients who complained to me of

excessive fatigue along with such other related problems as nervousness, depression, muscle and joint aches and pains, poor appetite, indigestion, irregular bowel habits, constipation, and irritability, all begin to feel better in a matter of only 48 hours with the administration of brewer's yeast. Their improvement was both sudden and dramatic. In only 5 days, all these secondary complaints disappeared completely.

Many of my patients have become so impressed with the efficacy of brewer's yeast that they use it as a quick and lasting energy pick-up instead of coffee, tea, or coke for the entire family—even including grandparents and grandchildren.

As Sandra L. told me, "My young teen-age daughter, Sue, no longer goes to the refrigerator for a coke when she needs an energy lift. Instead, she goes straight to the brewer's yeast jar whenever she feels even slightly fatigued while doing her homework. She stirs a heaping tablespoonful into orange juice or grape juice and drinks it down. Within a few minutes, she notices a definite physical and mental energy pick-up that lasts for several hours."

I'm sure you'll agree with me that when a teen-ager turns down a soft drink for brewer's yeast it must be good. Now let's find out just exactly . . .

**What This Potent
Energy Builder Can Do for You**

If you know what brewer's yeast consists of, you will better understand how it can help you so much in recovering your lost energy. So let's consider that point first.

Without a doubt, brewer's yeast is one of the most potent foods you can eat. It is loaded down with the entire vitamin B complex, 19 amino acids which make it a complete protein, and 18 minerals. Except for the absence of vitamins A, C, and E, it can be considered to be a whole food.

So if you're tired and worn-out all the time, if you have no pep or energy, if you wake up as tired as when you went to bed, if you drag around all day long—*and if your doctor has already ruled out any serious health problem*—then get yourself some brewer's yeast. It can do wonders for you. If the simple lack of energy is your only problem, you could feel a lot better in just a few short days.

You can get brewer's yeast in 3 different forms: flakes, pills, or powder. The yeast flakes have a milder flavor, but it takes more of them to give the equivalent of the powder. It also takes about 24 tablets to equal one tablespoon of yeast powder. So yeast powder is the best way to go.

Most of my patients who use brewer's yeast to gain energy start out with a teaspoonful of powder in fruit juice or tomato juice in the morning. As they become used to it, they increase the amount up to a tablespoonful. Then, throughout the day, whenever they begin to feel an energy lag, they take another spoonful of brewer's yeast, again, either in juice or hot bouillon.

I suggest that you do the same. A tablespoonful of brewer's yeast with each meal and at your mid-morning and mid-afternoon work breaks in place of coke or coffee will give you more energy to get things done than you ever thought possible before.

Brewer's yeast, like other protein foods, is high in phosphorus. So it is always wise to take extra calcium (one or 2,000 milligrams a day in the form of dolomite), because when excess phosphorus is excreted from the body it always pulls calcium out with it. I routinely ask my patients who are taking brewer's yeast to take dolomite to get that extra calcium they need. I prefer dolomite over bonemeal because, although bonemeal does contain calcium, it also contains phosphorus, and the average diet has an ample supply of it already.

How This Invigorating Food
Performed a Sexual Miracle for Freda C.

Wheat germ is a superior catalytic health energizer. It is an excellent food. A grain of wheat, like all seeds, contains the nutriment needed for germination and growth. Protein, minerals, the vitamin B complex, fats, and carbohydrates are all present in the proper proportions. The germ or embryo of the wheat kernel contains most of the vitamins and proteins of the highest quality.

Vitamin E is also present in high concentrations in the oil of the wheat germ.

That, basically, is the story of wheat germ. Now let me show you what wheat germ and its oil can do by telling you about Freda C's experience.

Freda was married when she was 18. Although her physical body was mature and she was fully developed sexually, she had never had any menstrual periods. Occasionally, there would be a bit of spotting, but there was nothing that even remotely resembled a normal monthly menstrual flow.

She and her husband, Paul, both wanted children; so she went to several specialists who gave her a variety of medications, hoping to help her conceive. But nothing ever happened. After 9 years of marriage without a pregnancy, Freda and Paul decided to give up and adopt a child.

However, at about this time, Freda happened to read an article in a health magazine about wheat germ and wheat germ oil helping infertile women to conceive. She asked her doctor about this, but his only response was to ridicule the idea as an "old wives' tale." With that, Freda decided to leave him and seek help from a doctor who used natural healing methods rather than drugs to cure their patients. That is why she came to my office.

I had Freda use wheat germ granules in almost everything she ate: soups, gravies, cereals, juices, hamburger, meat loaf, and so on. I also had her take one 20 minim wheat germ oil capsule with each meal.

Nothing out of the ordinary happened for 3 months. Then, for the first time in her life, Freda experienced a full normal menstrual flow.

Her menstrual periods continued every month for the next 5 months. Then, without warning, they stopped again. Freda was extremely disappointed and depressed over this situation.

About a month later, she became extremely nauseous every morning, but she attributed this to a bad case of the flu. However, when the flu was over, her nausea still remained; so I asked her to get a lab test for possible pregnancy. The test came back positive· Freda was pregnant.

Her baby, a healthy, husky, 7-1/2 pound boy, was born last summer. Freda regards wheat germ and wheat germ oil as a miracle food, and who can say it's not, for it certainly performed a sexual miracle for her.

How You Can Use This Miracle Health Food Yourself

As I told you in the beginning of this section, wheat germ is a superior catalytic health vitalizer. With its accompanying vitamin E, wheat germ is essential to health and well-being. Cattle, deprived of wheat germ and vitamin E, have dropped dead from heart disease while grazing in the pasture. Drs. Wilfrid and Evan Shute's work has proven its value in cardiac cases, for they have rehabilitated the hearts of thousands of people with the vitamin E from wheat germ. I'll tell you much more about that later on in Chapter 8.

Wheat germ oil has been tested in many scientific laboratories on both animals and people, especially athletes. It has been found to be invaluable in building energy and beating fatigue. You can use the granules and the capsules just as Freda did. Do so, and I know you'll agree with me that wheat germ is an outstanding catalytic health food to build up your pep and energy, your vigor and vitality.

How a "Medicine of the Future" Is Used to Cure Arthritis

I first heard of this amazing catalytic health vitalizer from Dave W. Dave had suffered for 8 years with rheumatoid arthritis. He had lived first on aspirin, then on cortisone, next Indocin, after that, Butazolidin, and so on, but his disease became progressively worse. He had quite a bit of crippling from his arthritis and was in constant, severe pain. He was unable to work; in fact, he was confined to bed most of the time.

Then a friend of Dave's father told him how he had cured his own arthritis by drinking alfalfa tea and taking alfalfa tablets.

Dave knew he had nothing to lose; he was now ready to try anything. He drank 4 cups of alfalfa tea and took 36 alfalfa tablets daily for 3 months. Slowly but surely the pain lessened and mobility returned to his joints. His general health also improved. His anemia disappeared, and he gained some badly needed weight.

Today, except for some painless, minor limitation of movement in his wrists and shoulders, Dave lives a completely normal, healthy life. He has gone back to work and is putting in 40 hours every week on his job. In fact, he sometimes even works overtime when he's needed.

Dave has also altered his diet a great deal in addition to using the alfalfa tea and tablets, which he continues to take. He no longer uses white sugar, coffee, highly processed foods, or white flour. He makes every effort to eat more fresh fruit and vegetables, bran and fiber, less meats but other protein rich foods. He feels that even if this diet has not helped his arthritis, it has definitely improved his general health.

As I've said previously, I've never been reluctant to learn from my patients; so I immediately tried out Dave's alfalfa remedy for arthritis. Let me give you the results I obtained in just a few short case histories.

1. ALFALFA USED TO CURE HAROLD C'S ARTHRITIS

Harold had been bothered off and on with rheumatism and arthritis in his back for a number of years. He got along by taking aspirin to kill most of the pain, but it finally got so bad that he could hardly get in and out of his car; so he came to see me.

A complete dietary analysis revealed no major vitamin or mineral deficiency in Harold's food intake; so I decided to have him take alfalfa, this marvelous catalytic health energizer Dave had told me about.

Harold drank alfalfa tea several times a day and also took alfalfa tablets, 12 of them 4 times a day, for a total of 48. The use of alfalfa worked wonderfully for Harold. In only a month his ex cruciating pains disappeared. Although the effects of his arthritis

59

can still be seen in his spinal x-rays, symptomatically Harold is well.

He still bowls in a senior citizens' league every week and goes around the golf course in the high 80's. Not bad for a 71 year old who could barely get in and out of his car a few months ago. Without a doubt, alfalfa is a terrific catalytic health energizer, no matter what a person's age or condition might be.

2. LEE AND MARY M. BOTH BENEFIT
FROM THIS WONDER FOOD

Lee and Mary were both troubled with arthritis. They had received no help whatever from their doctor's treatment. Mary's main problem was in her hands and wrists. They were extremely stiff and sore and painful when she worked. Her arthritis was slowly moving to her right elbow and shoulder, and she was afraid it might completely cripple her before it ran its course.

Lee's arthritis had settled mainly in the hips and knee joints. He walked with extreme difficulty, requiring a cane. Each step was painful misery to him.

As so often happens in cases where routine medical treatment gets no results, they began to read health books and magazines, trying to find the solution to their problem for themselves. They read about the alfalfa remedy and asked their doctor for his opinion.

"He practically laughed us out of his office," Lee said. "Made me feel like an idiot. Told me alfalfa was absolutely useless and had no therapeutic value whatever. When I asked him to read the article I had with me before he made up his mind, he said he had no time for such junk and refused. Said drugs were the only possible answer. But his drugs had never helped Mary or me; so we never went back to him again and we never will."

I told Lee and Mary to go ahead with the treatment the article had recommended: 4 cups of alfalfa tea each day. However, in addition to the tea I asked them to take 36 to 48 alfalfa tablets daily.

That was more than 10 years ago. Neither Lee nor Mary has had any sign of the arthritis that bothered them when they came to my office. Lee threw his cane away only 6 months after he started the treatment. Mary does her housework now with no pain or discomfort whatever in her hands and wrists. And they're no "spring chickens" by any means. They're both up their late 70's now, and getting along well in all respects.

The final ironic touch of their case history is this: The doctor who laughed Lee and Mary out of his office more than 10 years ago is no longer in active practice. He retired prematurely because he became stricken with a severe case of arthritis. He is now mainly confined to his home, going out only occasionally, and then only in a wheelchair.

3. HOW KEVIN F. OVERCAME
THIS PAINFUL, CRIPPLING DISEASE

Although we usually think of arthritis as being a disease of old age, this is not always true. Rheumatoid arthritis can attack at any age. The onset is usually abrupt with simultaneous inflammation of many joints and progressive involvement of new joints. Pain, tenderness, redness, heat, and swelling are the primary symptoms. Secondary symptoms include mental depression and excessive fatigue. Medical treatment usually consists of corticosteroids to fight the joint inflammation, but they can have extremely dangerous side effects.

Kevin F. was only 34 years old when he was stricken with extreme pain and swelling in his knees and ankles. He went immediately to an expert in this field, a medical doctor who specialized in rheumatology.

This doctor correctly diagnosed his condition as rheumatoid arthritis and prescribed drugs and hot baths for pain relief. As Kevin told me, he sat in the tub day after day in the hottest water he could stand while tears of pain poured down his face.

After 3 months of this futile treatment, Kevin gave up and came to me for help. He came into my office in a wheelchair, for his knees were so badly swollen he could not stand up because of the excruciating pain.

His condition was so severe that I frankly had my doubts about the ability of alfalfa to help him. But I asked him to try this treatment. I had him use my usual procedure of 4 cups of alfalfa tea daily and 12 alfalfa tablets 4 times a day for a total of 48.

In only 3 weeks Kevin's knees had returned almost to normal. The swelling was gone, and he could now stand up without pain in them. In 2 more months he went back to work and has never been troubled since. Kevin has literally been a *walking* advertisement for me and for alfalfa. He has sent scores of arthritis sufferers to my office to learn of this new treatment.

What Alfalfa Can Do for You

If you are troubled with arthritis or rheumatism that has not responded to any conventional treatment, why not try alfalfa? It has been found to provide resistance to many diseases. It seems to be especially helpful in those conditions that end in -*itis*, such as arthritis, neuritis, bronchitis, and the like.

Alfalfa also helps prevent fatigue and exhaustion, thus earning its title as a catalytic health vitalizer. This makes it of great value in fighting rheumatoid arthritis, for excessive fatigue is one of the secondary symptoms of the disease. As far as dosage for arthritis and rheumatism goes, I have always used at least twice the number of tablets recommended by the manufacturer on the bottle.

Alfalfa also has other healing properties that sometimes really amaze me. Wanda C. told me about the experience her husband had with it. Victor was literally allergic to spring, and when you're a farmer, as he was, that's really bad news.

Victor took medication to try to combat his allergies. These helped, but gradually they lost their potency as his body adjusted to them. Every spring he found himself constantly sneezing and gasping for air through a clogged-up nose. Sleep was almost impossible for him, and he dragged around all day red-eyed and bone-weary from the lack of rest.

Then Wanda read that alfalfa is sometimes good for colds and sinus conditions. Victor decided to try it. His problem was resolved almost overnight on only 6 tablets a day.

Wanda says her entire family—including 3 young children

under the age of 10—takes alfalfa tablets now, and they haven't had a cold or even a sniffle for ages.

Alfalfa is often used by leading vitamin manufacturing companies as a base for their multi-vitamin, multi-mineral tablets, for it is one of the most complete and nutritionally rich foods ever found. Not only does it have an exceptionally high level of vitamins and minerals, but it is also high in protein and contains every amino acid essential to a person's health. Its antitoxin or detoxification properties exceed those of liver, brewer's yeast, and wheat germ.

Alfalfa has all the fat-soluble vitamins—A, D, E, and K—as well as vitamin C and the entire B complex. Its minerals include phosphorus, calcium, potassium, sodium, chlorine, sulphur, magnesium, copper, manganese, and iron, as well as most of the trace minerals.

Dr. David Kritchevsky, Ph.D., a biochemist, and a former winner of the Borden Award of the American Institute of Nutrition, has been working with alfalfa for more than 10 years, studying its role in relation to coronary heart disease. Experiments he and his associates have performed in the laboratory indicate that alfalfa has the ability to lower high levels of chrolesterol. Dr. Kritchevsky thinks the potential value of alfalfa is so great that he says, "Alfalfa is the research wave of the future."

4

How a Specific Mineral Catalyzer Can Vitalize Your System and Restore Your Zest for Living

This mineral is truly one of nature's most potent catalytic health vitalizers. Not only can it cure specific ailments in the body, but it can also give you power and energy to spare. It supplies that vital spark to light the fires of energy that burn in your body.

You need no less than 16 specific mineral catalyzers to maintain your good health, lengthen and amplify your prime of life, and keep your energy reserves at a high level. However, I have devoted this chapter to the discussion of only one—calcium—for, according to nutritional authorities, the American diet is more lacking in it than in any other essential food. I have also found that to be true in my own practice.

A Deficiency of This Catalytic Health
Vitalizer Causes Premature Aging

If you lack sufficient calcium in your diet, you will age prematurely—growing old long before your time. Dr. Henry C. Sherman, the noted biochemist, has stated in effect that the prime period of human life could be extended by a moderate increase in calcium in the diet of those who are in or approaching the ranks of senior citizens.

I personally feel that an individual should not wait until he is old to start taking supplemental calcium. He should start taking from one to 2,000 milligrams of calcium in the form of dolomite when he is young, and he should keep up this good health habit all his life. It would also be wise to be sure to get at least 400 units of vitamin D daily to insure the proper absorption of calcium from the digestive tract into the body where it can be utilized.

The absence of this essential catalytic health energizer can cause you all sorts of trouble. Moreover, its addition to the diet will cure a number of ailments, as you will see in this chapter. For instance, I have used calcium successfully to alleviate hot flashes and other menstrual disorders. Let me give you just one such example:

How Dora R's Unbearable Hot Flashes
Were Eliminated Quickly and Easily

Dora came to me suffering with a severe problem of hot flashes. She had undergone a hysterectomy a few years before, and shortly after that her hot flashes had become almost unbearable. They were accompanied by profuse sweating, dizziness, and fatigue. They would often be followed by chills, a rapid and fluttering pulse and palpitations of the heart. Dora said it felt as if her heart was coming right up into her throat.

Her hands and feet would tingle and become numb. She asked her doctor what could be done about it, but he only shrugged off her problem by saying that this was a common ailment for women her age and she would just have to learn to live with it. Other than this useless advice, he offered no solution for her problem.

However, since Dora's condition was also interfering with her performance at work, she couldn't afford to "just live with it," so she came to me for help.

I have had great success in treating a large number of female patients who had this problem; the treatment involved the use of 800 to 1,200 units of vitamin E daily. I decided to use this same procedure for Dora. However, the numbness and tingling in her hands and feet and the rapid pulse and palpitations of her heart indicated she had some other dietary deficiency that could be contributing to her problem.

A complete analysis of her diet revealed exactly what I suspected: Dora was suffering from a severe calcium deficiency. I therefore recommended that she take 2,000 milligrams of calcium each day in the form of dolomite. Within the month, her hot flashes had been completely eliminated, except for a very mild flushing once or twice a day. This, too eventually disappeared with her continued use of dolomite and vitamin E.

Not only did Dora's hot flashes disappear, but her other symptoms—the dizziness and fatigue, the rapid pulse and palpitating heart, the numbness and tingling in her hands and feel—also vanished.

All in all, Dora says she feels a thousand percent better. She feels more alert and active than she has for many years. I am not at all surprised at her feeling of increased energy, for calcium is absolutely essential for a vigorous, healthy body and an active, alert mind.

How You Can Benefit from Dora's Experience

Certain conditions seem to bother us as we get older: for instance, prostate problems for men, hot flashes and other menopausal disorders for women. I have already discussed the male prostate problem, so let me now cover a woman's difficulty with hot flashes—one of the most troublesome ailments of the change of life and beyond that a woman has to put up with.

"A man will never understand this problem completely," Vivian Y. told me. "I used to have hot flashes so bad I actually thought I was going to physically suffocate. But my husband thought I was only exaggerating. Thank heaven your treatment of vitamin E and dolomite with its calcium solved this problem for me."

I would suggest the same remedy for you, too, if you are now suffering with those troublesome and irritating hot flashes. You can use 800 to 1,200 units of vitamin E along with enough dolomite tablets to get at least 2,000 milligrams of calcium each day. If you have high blood pressure or a past history of rheumatic heart disease, your vitamin E treatment should be initiated slowly and cautiously. No more than 100 units a day should be taken in the beginning.

Let me explain the reason for this more fully. Vitamin E will not hurt you; it is not dangerous as so many drugs are. It is, however, so efficient in strengthening your heart muscle that a stronger and firmer heart beat may cause the blood pressure to rise slightly higher for a short period of time.

In the case of a history of rheumatic heart disease where part of the heart has been left weaker and scarred—causing an imbalance of the heart beat—the vitamin E can improve the healthy part of the heart so dramatically that it can temporarily increase the imbalance even further.

If you are in any doubt about taking vitamin E, ask your doctor. It would be wise, however, to ask one who is aware of the capabilities of vitamin E, rather than one who believes only in drug therapy.

I have always recommended at least 2,000 milligrams per day of calcium for my female patients with menopausal symptoms or hot flashes, for calcium does much to relieve pain and relax muscular and nervous tension. This amount may seem high to you, but as I've said before, when calcium is taken in the form of dolomite, where it is in its natural combination with magnesium, there is no possibility of an overdose. For older patients, who have trouble with the absorption of calcium from the digestive tract, I have used as much as 4 to 5 thousand milligrams daily to get favorable results.

I can assure you that you will feel much better with the use of vitamin E and dolomite. Not only will your hot flashes be terminated or lessened, but you'll have more vim and vigor, pep, energy, and vitality to meet the daily strains and stresses of modern living, for calcium is an extremely potent catalytic health vitalizer.

Other Benefits You Can Gain from This Marvelous Catalytic Health Vitalizer

Calcium in the form of dolomite is also useful for a variety of other ailments. It can be used as a calming and sedative agent to help cure insomnia. The value at bedtime of the proverbial glass of warm milk to help one get to sleep is attributed to its calcium content.

An adequate supply of calcium is necessary for proper functioning of the digestive tract. Spasms in the intestine—many times mistaken for colitis—and spastic constipation are often alleviated by an increase of calcium in the diet.

This catalytic health energizer is also highly useful as a pain killer. Calcium injections have been used for the pains of pleurisy and migraine headaches. It is also effective in reducing the pain of broken bones. I have seen calcium soothe arthritis and rheumatic pains in as little as 1 to 3 days. Oral calcium can be used for labor pains, muscular aches, and stomach cramps. Let me give you several examples now so you can see for yourself how this catalytic health vitalizer can be useful in so many different kinds of situations.

How I Used This Mineral Catalyzer to Cure Gail D's Sore and Painful Breasts

Gail had been bothered for 5 years with extremely sore and painful breasts about a week or 10 days before each menstrual period. Her breasts were so sore and tender she could not even sleep on her stomach.

After a complete dietary analysis, I found that Gail was extremely deficient in calcium, so I placed her on 2,500 milligrams of calcium a day in the form of dolomite. Her relief was dramatic and immediate. The very next menstrual period arrived without being preceded by the sore and painful breasts that had always plagued her before.

Last fall Gail and her husband, Lewis, went on a 3 week camping trip in Canada. Unfortunately, Gail forgot to take along her dolomite. She had her menstrual period during that time and she spent a miserable week before the flow actually started. As she told me when she got back, "Was I ever sorry I forgot my calcium . . . the pain in my breasts was just as bad as it was before. I'd almost forgot how bad it could be. I guarantee I'll never forget my dolomite again."

Gail's experience emphasizes a point that's well worth keeping in mind, and that is that vitamins, minerals, and other catalytic health energizers are always needed by the body. They are not like drugs in this respect. If you find that a certain catalytic health energizer such as calcium is needed to cure your ailment, maintain your good health, and build up your energy, then don't stop taking it just as soon as you feel better. You'll need to continue taking it every day the same way you need food and water, sleep and rest.

How Kenneth O's Elbow Pains Disappeared As if by Magic

Kenneth had been troubled with extreme pain in his right elbow for more than 2 years. At times, the pain was so severe he would not be able to work, for he was able to use only his left arm. Any movement of his right arm during these acute attacks made the pain almost unbearable.

Kenneth's regular family doctor was not able to help him, so he sent Kenneth to a bone specialist. This doctor took all kinds of x-rays of Kenneth's elbow, ran a variety of laboratory tests, and in the final report with Kenneth, he said, "I can find nothing at all wrong with your elbow." When Kenneth insisted there had to be something wrong somewhere, this specialist finally said, "Well, if you still think you're sick, maybe you'd better see a psychiatrist." As Kenneth told me, "That was the last straw; that did it," and he came to my office.

I, too, x-rayed Kenneth's elbow and found only some minor arthritic changes which by themselves were not enough to cause the extreme pain he suffered. I then x-rayed his cervical spine to look for some bone spurs or possible nerve irritation caused by vertebral impingement, but again, I found nothing sufficient to warrant his severe pain.

Next came a complete analysis of the mineral intake in his diet. There I found the culprit: insufficient calcium. I started Kenneth immediately on 3,000 milligrams of calcium in the form of dolomite. I also gave him 400 units of vitamin D each day to make sure the calcium would be properly absorbed. In addition to the vitamin D, I had Kenneth take 5,000 milligrams of vitamin C. I have found that vitamin C is valuable in speeding up the healing processes in cases of arthritis, bursitis, and rheumatism.

In less than 10 days, Kenneth's elbow pains disappeared as if by magic. He got along fine for 6 months with no trouble whatever, and then, as so often happens with a lot of us when the pain is gone, Kenneth forgot to follow the doctor's advice and failed to take his "medicine." His elbow pains came back literally overnight and for a fleeting moment he couldn't understand why. Then he remembered he had failed to come back for more dolomite when he ran out.

Just as soon as he resumed taking the dolomite again, the pains vanished. Kenneth's case is simply another example of the necessity of continuing to take the catalytic health energizer that solves your problem. For example, Kenneth's body will never lose its need for calcium. Nor will yours or mine, for that matter.

How This Amazing Catalytic Health Vitalizer Cured Marlene A's Neck Arthritis

I never cease to be amazed at the abysmal lack of knowledge of some of the members of the healing arts when it comes to the use of nutrition to cure disease. Of course, I realize that both the medical colleges and the nursing schools give scant attention to nutritional therapy. For instance, take Marlene A. She is a registered nurse who works for an ophthalmologist specializing in eye surgery.

Marlene had been plagued with arthritis in the neck for many years. She blamed it on her occupational position, for she was bending over a surgical table 5 to 6 hours every day assisting in eye surgery. She also had constant pain in her lower back, again presumably from the same reason. Her employer also had the same problems with which Marlene suffered.

Finally, it reached the point where Marlene could no longer stand the pain in her neck and lower back, so she sought help from a specialist in rheumatic and arthritic diseases. This gentleman recommended a lower back brace and a cervical collar for Marlene, but this did little to help her.

She finally came to me in despair and as a last resort, for it is sometimes difficult for nurses and medical doctors to accept a chiropractor as a valid practitioner of the healing arts. X-rays of Marlene's neck revealed bony spurs and calcium deposits at the 4th and 5th cervical levels and some calcification in the lumbar area in the small of the back.

It was difficult for Marlene to understand that she had insufficient calcium in her diet when these calcium deposits were present in her x-rays, but she was ready to try anything. I asked her to take 2,000 milligrams of calcium each day in the form of dolomite along with 800 units of vitamin D and 5,000 milligrams of vitamin C.

In only a week Marlene called to say that her pain was 50 percent better, both in her neck and her lower back. In less than a month, she was completely without pain.

Marlene's case had a domino effect. When her employer saw how much better she was, he, too, decided to try dolomite along with the vitamins D and C. He had been using traction, muscle relaxing drugs, and various pain killers when he started the dolomite treatment. At the end of only 10 days, he was so much better he could hardly believe it. He stopped using all the other drugs and stayed only with the dolomite and vitamins. Within 3 months he had forgotten that he ever had any problems at all.

His wife, who also suffered a great deal with rheumatic aches and pains in her knees and hips, also decided to try the dolomite "medicine," as she called it. She, too, was quickly relieved of her painful ailment.

And to top it off, Marlene's husband, a city bus driver who was troubled constantly with pain in his upper dorsals and shoulders from his job, also decided to try dolomite and vitamins C and D. He had been taking aspirin and using sleeping pills in an attempt to get some rest each night. In less than a month, Marlene said he was sleeping like a baby. He went to work with a smile each morning instead of dreading to get up as he had before.

Why Extra Calcium Was Needed in All These Cases

Let me explain something here about why calcium spurs and deposits are indications of insufficient calcium in the diet. You see, when the body does not get enough calcium, it will withdraw what little calcium it has from the bones to make sure there is enough in the bloodstream. There calcium is absolutely necessary for the healing of wounds, clotting of blood, the stimulation of certain enzyme action, and control of the passage of body fluids through the cells and tissue walls. The proper amount of calcium in the blood is also needed for proper nervous activity and for normal contraction and relaxation of the heart muscle.

As the calcium is withdrawn from the bones to do this work, the body's innate intelligence does its best to bolster the sagging body architecture, and it starts building bony deposits and spurs to reduce movement and limit activity. It patches here and there the best it can, for it knows there is not enough calcium to rebuild the entire structure as it should be.

So you see, even with an insufficient calcium intake, you can have calcium deposits and bony spurs along with thin, porous, easily breakable bones (osteoporosis) all at the same time. And that's why more calcium—not less—is needed in the diet in cases of arthritis and rheumatism.

How Katherine O's Insomnia Was Resolved in Short Order with No More Sleeping Pills

Katherine was an extremely nervous, jumpy, and high-strung woman when she came to see me. She had been living on sedatives and tranquilizers which her previous doctor had prescribed for her. However, she eventually needed more and more and finally reached the point where these drugs were no longer effective for her. But her doctor refused to increase the dosage.

Katherine was really at wit's end; she did not know where to turn. A friend of hers suggested that she try some natural remedies for a change, and the friend gave Katherine a health magazine to read. In it Katherine found an article that told how sedatives, tranquilizers, and sleeping pills were not only completely worthless, but also highly dangerous as well. So Katherine decided to take a completely different approach to her nervous problem and ended up in my office.

My physical examination of Katherine revealed no specific physical difficulty that could be causing her insomnia. Nor was I able to discover any psychological or mental problems that could be a causative factor for her insomnia. There were no financial problems for her to worry about, as her husband was a highly successful businessman. She was suffering from some digestive problems as a result of all the drugs she'd been taking, but I felt sure these would clear up as soon as she got off her pill-popping habits.

After I ran a complete analysis of Katherine's dietary intake, I knew I had isolated her problem. As with so many insomniacs, Katherine was highly deficient in calcium. I immediately placed her on 3,000 milligrams of calcium a day in the form of dolomite along with 1,200 units of vitamin D. I also asked her to take 30 milligrams of zinc each day. Zinc is a natural tranquilizer for the nervous system.

In addition to this, I had Katherine take 6 tablets of calcium lactate before going to bed with a glass of warm milk. The calcium in calcium lactate is quickly and easily assimilated by the body; I have found it to be the best form to use just before going to bed for insomnia.

The very next night Katherine slept better than she ever had with all her sleeping pills. During the following weeks her body completely eliminated all the bad effects of the drugs in her sedatives and sleeping pills—this helped her natural remedies of calcium, vitamin D, and zinc to be even more effective. Katherine no longer has a bit of trouble sleeping. She tells me she has not slept this well since she was a small child. And sleep has done wonders for her both mentally and physically. The tired lines are gone from her face. She is full of pep and energy, and seems never to tire any more in the daytime.

I have since reduced her calcium intake to 2,000 milligrams and her vitamin D to 400 units daily. I have, however, left her zinc intake the same, 30 milligrams a day.

Before I finish this chapter, I would like to cover briefly several kinds of problems this catalytic health vitalizer can solve.

1. *Broken Bones Will Not Heal Properly Without Calcium.* My niece, Carla L., who lives in the midwest, broke her leg over a year ago. She had been under a doctor's care there, but the break did not heal properly and was still extremely painful to her. Her mother wrote to me and said they were spending a lot of money on vitamins and physiotherapy for Carla, but without results. Her leg still hurt her a great deal. She was also drinking a quart of milk a day, but that hadn't seemed to help either.

I wrote to Carla's mother and told her that all the vitamins in the world wouldn't help unless Carla had enough calcium in her diet to heal the broken bone. I suggested that she have Carla take 3,000 milligrams of calcium a day in the form of dolomite and told her if that didn't help, I'd pay for the dolomite myself.

A month later I got a letter from Carla herself. She said she had thrown away her crutches and was walking now without any pain and only the slightest suggestion of a limp. Another letter 6 weeks later said she was completely back to normal again.

2. *How Calcium Can Help Tic Douloureux.* I received a letter from a former patient of mine, Nina T., who now lives in California. Her mother had suffered with facial neuralgia or tic douloureux for many years. After Nina had got rid of her own nervous problem with dolomite, she asked her mother to try it for her ailment. Her mother's condition disappeared in a week. It never returned except once when she was hospitalized and could not take her dolomite. As soon as she was out of the hospital and resumed her dolomite "medication," her facial neuralgia again vanished.

3. *How This Catalytic Health Vitalizer Relieves Growing Pains.* Mrs. Velma P. wrote me to tell of her young son's experience with dolomite and how it had healed his growing pains.

"I read about that boy, Hal, and his growing pains in your book, *Extraordinary Healing Secrets*, and how dolomite helped him, so we decided to try it on our 10 year old son, Joel, who had the same problem."

Velma said they did just what I reported in my book. They crushed half a dozen dolomite tablets in a glass of milk and Joel drank it before he went to bed. He slept all night and never woke up once. Always before, his mother had been up several times a night to rub his legs. He now takes 1,000 milligrams every day and it's been more than 3 months without a single sign of his previous pains.

4. *How Calcium Can Cure Brittle Fingernails.* If you have a problem with brittle fingernails that are constantly breaking off, then the case history of Connie N. will be of interest to you.

Connie's nails would peel off in layers. They were brittle and broke easily and she was always snagging them on her clothes. She had tried gelatin capsules to strengthen them but without success.

I had her take 2,000 milligrams of calcium every day. In less than 3 months her fingernails were strong and flexible again. If you don't have this problem, this case history may not seem like a big deal to you. But if you do have this trouble, you'll understand quite well why it's here for you to read.

5. *How This Catalytic Health Vitalizer Helped an Entire*

Family. I gave a patient of mine, Joy S., some dolomite tablets for her pre-menstrual tension and severe cramps. They worked so well for her she soon had her entire family taking dolomite.

She says it helps her husband relax and get to sleep as soon as he goes to bed. Before he used to roll and toss for a couple of hours. Her younger son, 9 year old Chris, used to suffer with leg cramps and pain in his feet. Since taking dolomite, he no longer has this problem.

Joy says that dental bills have become almost non-existent for them since they've been taking dolomite. Their dentist says that they have the healthiest looking teeth and gums that he's seen in a long time. What terrific "medicine" dolomite with its calcium is.

Three important mineral catalytic health vitalizers I have not discussed in this chapter are zinc, potassium, and iron. I have already mentioned the use of zinc in prostate problems in Chapter 2. I will cover its healing capabilities in skin conditions, infections, and nervous ailments in later chapters where it is more appropriate. The use of potassium will be discussed in Chapter 13. I am not going to talk about the mineral catalyzer, iron, in this book because so much information is available everywhere, and it seemed too repetitious to me. My omission of iron does not imply that it is not important to a person's health; it is.

5

How to Solve Embarrassing and Troublesome Skin Problems Without Dangerous Drugs or Expensive Medicines

Skin conditions, such as acne, eczmea, rashes, warts, psoriasis, even dandruff, are embarrassing nuisances to the individual. Sometimes, as with certain kinds of eczema, these skin problems are more than an inconvenience, for they can become sore and painful and actually interfere with job performance or ordinary, everyday living. In some cases, there is also the added risk of dangerous infection.

In addition, skin conditions cause a definite loss of energy. Whenever the human body is sick, it always takes energy to heal it. Skin conditions are no exception. At times, this physical loss of energy is augmented by the patient's mental attitude toward his problem. The first case history, which I'll discuss in just a few moments, is a special example of that.

A negative mental attitude just by itself can cause a definite loss of energy. I have seen patients with skin problems drag into my waiting room, slump and slouch down in a corner away from a light, and try to hide behind a newspaper or magazine because of embarrassment about their ailment.

I have also seen these same patients, completely cured of their skin problems, come bounding into the office, smiling and happy, full of energy and vitality, ready to take on the world.

Most of my patients with skin problems had already been the route of the skin specialist without success. They had medicine cabinets at home filled with useless salves, ointments, and lotions that had failed to work.

So if you have any sort of skin condition that has not healed—acne, a rash, warts, eczema, psoriasis, even dandruff—don't give up hope, even if you feel you have exhausted all the orthodox medical possibilities of a cure.

Keep right on reading this chapter. It could well be that you will find the answer to your own individual problem right here in these pages. I can assure you of one thing: none of the catalytic health vitalizers you'll find here will ever hurt you or make your condition worse. They can only help you.

Now for the first case history. I have gone into much more detail in this one than I usually do, for I wanted you to see just how much a skin condition can affect an individual mentally and emotionally, and how it can drastically change a person's life.

**How Thelma Z's Complexion Problem
Was Finally Solved with This
Exceptional Catalytic Health Vitalizer**

Thelma had suffered with an acne problem since she was 13 years old. As most young people do, she accepted this as a teen-age curse which would pass when she became older, although she did try a variety of over-the-counter remedies which she had seen advertised on TV or in teen-age magazines. None of these helped her—which is "par for the course" for these highly promoted, but useless medications.

However, her condition did not disappear as she had hoped it would. Unfortunately, when she was 20, her problem became much worse. Not only her face, but also her back and chest were covered with pimples in all stages of development. Even her buttocks were broken out, and it was often painful for her to sit down. Her thighs and legs were not broken out, but they were always extremely rough and scaly and appeared to be covered with goose bumps.

Thelma was so embarrassed and ashamed of her condition that she no longer wanted to date and became more and more withdrawn from society. She quit her position as a sales clerk because she thought people were staring at her. She then took a job as a night telephone operator from 11 PM to 7 AM for a physicians' answering service. As soon as she got off work, she went straight to her apartment and stayed there all day with the blinds tightly drawn. She went out only to get groceries, go to work, and occasionally to see a movie.

Finally, Thelma's mother convinced her that she could not spend the rest of her life that way and got her to go to a dermatologist for help. This doctor prescribed tetracycline for her, an oral antibiotic that is often used for acne. However, he gave Thelma a nonrenewable prescription for only a 30 day supply of Achromycin V, one of the most expensive forms of tetracycline. This meant Thelma had to return to him every month to get her prescription renewed.

Thelma followed this procedure for nearly 2 years, but she achieved no lasting results. Finally, one day she asked the doctor exactly how long this treatment was going to last. He told her she would have to keep it up until her menopause!

Thelma never went back after that day; that was her last appointment. As she told me, she was not about to be drug dependent for 25 to 30 years. Not only that, but she was beginning to develop some bad side effects from the tetracycline. She now had

81

a severe case of vaginitis, which is not at all uncommon with this drug. Her stomach was also upset; she was suffering with a lot of gas and some diarrhea from its use.

Next Thelma set out on her own to see if she could cure herself. She eliminated almost all junk foods from her diet, and began taking multi-vitamin tablets along with some calcium and iron. This self-help program lasted for 6 months. Her condition improved slightly, but it was not completely resolved.

Finally, on the advice of a friend, she came to my office. I ran a mineral analysis of her diet and found, not at all to my surprise, that she was badly in need of zinc. I gave her only 30 milligrams a day in the form of zinc gluconate. How well did that work? Well, I'll let you judge the results for yourself.

In only 10 weeks, Thelma's complexion was completely changed for the better. Gone were the acne from her back and chest and the pimples from her buttocks. Her legs were no longer rough and scaly, nor did they have the appearance of goose bumps. Her face was radiant and glowing with happiness, for her complexion was clear, smooth, and beautiful. She no longer had any of the troublesome side effects of the tetracycline medication.

Her new appearance has changed Thelma's entire outlook on life. She quit her night job and is now working for a large department store in the women's clothing department. She is continuing her education by taking college night courses in sales and marketing, although as she told me on her last visit, some of this may have to change. It seems that she has developed a new interest in life; not just a man, but specifically *that certain man*.

How Mike D's Acne Was Marvelously Healed After Years of Embarrassment and Discomfort

Mike had acne from the time he was 12 until he was 25, 13 long years. Nothing had ever helped before he came to me. For the last several years, he had been going to a skin specialist for sunlamp treatments, injections, and a prescription for an ointment. Although this treatment helped keep Mike's acne under control, it did not cure it.

A friend of his, Allen W., who came to me for the same problem (which had been resolved), convinced Mike to come to my office for treatment. I found him to be deficient in zinc, as so many people with skin conditions are; so I placed him on 30 milligrams of zinc gluconate daily.

Within only 5 weeks Mike's complexion had cleared. He now has no sign of a pimple at all. He looks in the mirror each morning expecting to see some, but none have shown up. As Mike says, he really can't believe yet how good his face looks now, but the compliments he hears from his friends are positive proof.

Incurable Psoriasis Cleared Up
for Nick J. After 8 Long Years

Psoriasis is usually considered to be a completely incurable disease. Nick had suffered with it for 8 long years. He had scaly patches of it scattered in various spots from his scalp down to his knees. The most troublesome areas were on the back of his neck and around his elbows. Because of it, Nick could not wear a tight fitting collar or a tie. Nor could he wear a long sleeved shirt. There were also areas on his abdomen that itched horribly when he became hot and perspired heavily.

Nick had visited numerous doctors during this 8 year period, including several dermatologists. He had been given any number of prescriptions for creams, lotions, astringents, salves, and ointments, all of which he had used without such success. One dermatologist had used a cortisone cream which removed some of the scabs temporarily, but it did nothing more than that.

When Nick came to me, I frankly was at somewhat of a loss as to how to proceed, for I could find no definite vitamin or mineral deficiency in his diet. I also knew from my college textbooks that psoriasis was a so-called "incurable" disease. I did consider the use of vitamin E oil, but Nick told me he had already tried that and it had not helped him very much.

Some nutritional research I had done with lecithin indicated it could be valuable in the treatment of psoriasis; so I decided on this, for I knew it would not hurt Nick in any way.

I had him take 3 nineteen-grain lecithin capsules with each meal. Amazingly, in slightly less than 3 months, Nick's patches of psoriasis had disappeared. He was astounded at this, and to tell the truth, so was I. I had not expected such spectacular results, for psoriasis is one of those conditions that is stubborn beyond imagination.

After 6 months of taking 9 lecithin capsules every day and no longer suffering with psoriasis, Nick began to have second thoughts about continuing this treatment. So he stopped. Within less than a month, red scaly patches began to appear on his body exactly where they had been before. He immediately started taking the lecithin capsules again, and the psoriasis vanished once more.

Nick no longer has any doubts as to what has cured his ailment. Nor does he have any desire to experiment again. He is perfectly content to accept things the way they are and not fight the problem. As he says, 9 lecithin capsules a day is a small price to pay for good health.

Twenty Years of Misery Ended for Gary B.

Not long after I had taken care of Nick's psoriasis, Gary B. came to me with a back problem. He also had psoriasis and had accepted it as an incurable condition, for he'd had it for more than 20 years.

The scaly red patches of his psoriasis were located mainly on his hands, arms, and scalp. I told Gary about Nick's experience and asked him if he would like to try some lecithin capsules himself.

Gary readily agreed and took the same amount Nick had, three 19 grain capsules 3 times a day. In addition to this, Gary sprinkled lecithin granules on his cereals and mixed it in his fruit juices. In 2 months, the scaly patches on his hands, arms, and scalp disappeared just as Nick's had done.

His wife, Lois, and his children were overjoyed for Gary. Lois called me the other day to say that for the first time in 20 years she could actually see nice clean clear skin on her husband's hands and arms. She was ever so happy for him.

Willis N. Makes a Phenomenal Recovery from Severe Burns Suffered in a Car Accident

Willis N's right hand was badly burned in a car accident. He had suffered both second and third degree burns, and his skin in places looked almost like charred elephant or rhinoceros hide. His physician had told Willis that some of the areas would have to be treated by skin grafts to prevent permanent disfiguration and crippling of his hand.

Willis had been a patient of mine for a long time; so he came to me for advice, too. I had him use vitamin E oil liberally on his hand each day. I also asked him to take 1,200 units of vitamin E internally. In addition to the vitamin E treatment, he soaked his hand 3 times a day in sterile water to which rose hip powder and granular vitamin C had been added.

We continued this treatment for 3 weeks after the accident and saw steady improvement each day. When Willis went back to the surgeon to discuss the skin grafts, he was told that his hand had improved so miraculously that surgery was no longer necessary.

He was in my office again the other day, 6 months after the accident, and except for a slight rosy color, his hand appears to be perfectly normal. I have no doubt that the color of his hand will be exactly as it was before the accident in just a few more months with his continued use of that phenomenal catalytic health vitalizer, vitamin E.

How This Exceptional Catalytic Health Vitalizer Healed Diabetic Skin Ulcers for Brenda F's Mother

Brenda F. is a patient of mine. Her mother is diabetic, and she had developed a badly ulcerated foot. After 3 weeks in the hospital, the doctor said it would not heal and wanted to amputate her foot just above the ankle.

Brenda's mother said absolutely not, refused further treatment, and left the hospital over the doctor's objections. Brenda brought her mother to me, knowing the success I'd had in treating skin conditions with vitamin E. I gave her mother 1,600 units of vitamin E daily. After 5 days, the vitamin E had improved the circulation so much that the blood started flowing in her foot again and the ulcer began to heal.

Although it took several more weeks, in the end the ulcer healed completely and her foot returned to normal. This exceptional catalytic health energizer allowed Brenda's mother to save her foot and avoid needless surgery that would have crippled her for the rest of her life.

How This Catalytic Health Vitalizer Can Magically Heal Scar Tissue

The son of one of my patients had a bad accident in the swimming pool the summer before last. He was 8 years old at the time and an excellent swimmer. However, he was over-confident in his abilities to dive. He did a back flip off the edge of the pool and instead of coming down in the water, he caught his forehead on the edge of the decking.

He split the skin on his forehead at a slant running from just above the left eyebrow up to the right temple. Thirty-two stitches were required to close the cut. Kathleen brought Ellis to me to see if I could do anything about the fiery red, long sweeping scar.

I told Kathleen to massage the scar every night with the oil from a 400 unit vitamin E capsule and to keep this up indefinitely. Kathleen did this faithfully for 4 months and then brought Ellis back to the office so I could see him again.

I could hardly find the scar, even though I knew where it was. It was now so flat and unnoticeable that unless you knew exactly where to look, you would not realize it was there. The red and fiery color was completely gone.

Vitamin E is also useful to heal and fill in the scars of chicken pox and the scars of teen-age acne or any type of facial scar that is embarrassing to the individual.

For instance, a patient of mine, Charlie M., told me that when his wife, Arline, was in an auto accident, her face was so badly cut and sore from shattered windshield glass that she could not even wash it. So she applied vitamin E ointment liberally instead. Within 7 days, her face was healed with no scarring whatever.

Even the stretch marks of pregnancy can be eliminated or made much less obvious by the use of vitamin E, both externally and internally.

Other Uses I've Found for This Amazing Catalytic Health Vitalizer

1. HOW LUCY R'S FUNGUS INFECTION WAS HEALED WITH SPECTACULAR RESULTS

Several years ago Lucy developed a chronic fungus infection under the toenails on her right foot. Her toenails turned black as if they were dead. There was a rotten-smelling sticky exudate that seeped out from under the toenails. The flesh under them became thickened and was extremely tender. Then several of the toenails came off. Lucy's toes were so sore and tender that she could not wear a shoe on her right foot unless it was a sandal style, open at the end. Even the weight of a sheet or blanket at night hurt her.

Lucy tried a variety of topical salves and ointments that did not help. She soaked her feet in a variety of solutions that are often used for the fungus of athlete's foot, but to no avail.

When I asked her to try vitamin E oil from the 100 unit capsule, she said, "Why not? I've tried everything else!" She rubbed the vitamin oil on her toes every night when she went to bed and wore a white sock to protect her foot. She also massaged a light coating of vitamin E oil on her toes several times throughout the day.

The results were little short of miraculous. The black foul-smelling exudate stopped; the thickened skin disappeared; and her toenails grew back. Three months later, her feet were completely normal again.

87

2. ANNA C. MAKES HER SON'S
DIAPER RASH DISAPPEAR AS IF BY MAGIC

Anna had been my patient for a back problem before her son was born. Her pregnancy helped to straighten her spine, and I had not seen her in the office for some time, although we saw each other occasionally in the store or the restaurant.

She called me one day to ask if I could recommend something for her one year old son's diaper rash. She had tried various kinds of ointments that her pediatrician had advised, but none of them had helped. I told her to use vitamin E oil from the 400 unit capsule and rub it into the affected areas at each diaper change.

I forgot all about her problem until she called again a couple of weeks later. Anna said her son's diaper rash disappeared in a matter of 3 days, but to play it safe, she continued the treatment for over a week.

But this was not the main reason Anna called me. After her son was born, she had developed a rash on the ring finger of her left hand that had spread to the palm. She had quit wearing her rings and was using plastic gloves to wash dishes.

But since she'd been using vitamin E oil on her son's bottom, her hand had healed, too. She no longer had any sign of the rash that had plagued her for so long on her fingers and the palm of her hand.

3. ANOTHER USE FOR THIS
VERSATILE CATALYTIC HEALTH VITALIZER

I have used vitamin E successfully in case after case to rid patients of painful and troublesome warts. Many of these patients had been to dermatologists and had tried many salves, ointments, and lotions without success.

Most of us can put up with warts unless they are in places where they get bumped or scraped so that they become sore and tender or bleed. Plantar warts can be especially troublesome if the person has to be on his feet all day. One patient of mine, a letter carrier, had all the warts on his feet removed by surgery, but they grew back again. I gave him 1,200 units of vitamin E daily, internally, and he also rubbed vitamin E oil on the soles of his feet each day. In only 90 days, his warts were gone.

Facial warts can be especially distressing. One of my patients, Imogene B., was troubled with several large warts on her chin. I had her take 1,200 units of vitamin E orally, and we placed circular Band-aids that had been soaked in vitamin E oil over each wart. It took nearly 6 months, but at the end of that time, the warts were gone.

Garden Remedy Heals Skin Infection for Teresa V. with Superb Success

Most people living in Florida have some aloe vera growing in the backyard, for they know how valuable this plant can be for minor burns, sunburn, cuts, scrapes, poison ivy, even diaper rash. Aloe vera really has no limits for its use in skin conditions, as I learned from one of my readers.

Teresa wrote me to say that she had contracted a bad skin rash on the palm of her right hand from pressing down citrus fruits in an electric juicer. The skin on her hand cracked, peeled, and itched so badly that she went to a dermatologist for treatment. He used x-ray on her hand and prescribed an expensive lotion for her.

After she had used up the lotion, her condition was a little better; so she went back to him. He treated her hand with x-ray again and prescribed another more expensive lotion. When that had been used up, a total of 3 months had elapsed and Teresa was still a long way from being cured.

Then she happened to think of the aloe vera growing in her own backyard and decided to try it. She smeared the aloe gel on her hands 3 or 4 times a day. She put an especially heavy coating of it on at night and wore a loose fitting white glove to bed. Her hand improved immediately. In only 10 days the rash had disappeared altogether. "I could kick myself when I think of the money I wasted on that dermatologist!" Teresa said.

You do not have to live in Florida or any other tropical area to use aloe vera. You can buy it in a bottled form from any good health food store.

Determining Your Own Treatment for Skin Conditions

Let me cover briefly for you what you—or anyone in your family, for that matter—can use if you suffer from any of the following skin conditions:

Acne	Zinc gluconate
Bed sores	Lecithin
Burns, minor	Zinc gluconate
Dandruff	Zinc gluconate
Diaper rash	Vitamin E, lecithin, aloe vera
Eczema	Zinc gluconate
Fungus infection	Vitamin E
Poison ivy (oak)	Vitamin E and aloe vera
Psoriasis	Lecithin
Rash on hands	Vitamin E and aloe vera
Scar tissue	Vitamin E
Skin ulcers	Vitamin E
Sun burn	Vitamin E and aloe vera
Warts	Vitamin E

In the preceding table, aloe vera is meant to be used externally, zinc gluconate internally. However, when using vitamin E and lecithin, you can use them orally as well as externally for faster results. You can take from 1 to 3 lecithin capsules with each meal. Three or 4 hundred units of vitamin E per day should be sufficient, for skin conditions do not normally require the large amount of vitamin E that is indicated in other ailments, such as heart disease, for example. However, if you do not get results with that amount, simply increase the dosage to as high as 1,200 units per day, keeping in mind the previous precautions I have mentioned for high blood pressure and past rheumatic heart disease.

In addition to these catalytic health vitalizers, you would be wise to take a good multi-vitamin, multi-mineral tablet daily. You especially need lots of vitamin A to help prevent the scarring that can accompany acne.

Vitamin E as indicated in the table above is useful in helping to soften and heal scar tissue that is already present, but vitamin A can be of great assistance as a preventive measure to keep the scar from forming, especially in teen-age acne. If vitamin A is not used and teen-age acne has left facial scars, then vitamin E ointment applied regularly will actually fill in those scars, often to the point where they are no longer visible, or at least, barely discernible. Vitamin C is important in helping to prevent the skin condition from becoming badly infected.

The specific items indicated above for use in certain conditions are a result of my own personal experience in my practice. You may have slightly different metabolic requirements. After all, no two of us are ever exactly alike. In short, let's say you have acne that does not respond completely to zinc gluconate. Then you should try lecithin, vitamin E, and aloe vera, until you find out which one is best for you.

You might even need *lactobacillus acidophilus capsules*, which I have found to be helpful when nothing else worked for the patient. If you do use acidophilus, I would suggest that you use twice the amount recommended on the bottle by the manufacturer. His recommendations are for the nutritional requirements of a healthy person. You are using it for a sick body to cure a specific ailment.

In addition to lecithin and vitamin E, you can take 30 milligrams of zinc gluconate every day with all these conditions, for zinc is known to speed up the body's healing processes. In fact, it is always a good idea to add zinc to your diet in any condition, even when you are in apparently good health, for 8 out of every 10 Americans have a zinc deficiency.

I also wanted to mention something more about burns here. You should never try to treat severe 2nd and 3rd degree burns at home. There is always too much danger of an infection. However, minor burns that do not cover too large a skin surface or that do not have extensive weeping areas can be safely treated. Vitamin E is also useful in reducing the redness and scar tissue and· in otherwise restoring the skin to normal in cases of large severe burns requiring extensive medical treatment, *after the skin has healed over and is no longer weeping a fluid exudate.*

To use vitamin E or lecithin externally, simply make a pinhole in the end of the capsule and squeeze out the liquid. I always use the capsules containing 400 international units of vitamin E, for even though they are more expensive than those containing 100, 200, or 300 units, they are the most potent. Vitamin E for external use also comes in the form of a cream or ointment. This is fine for skin maintenance *after the acute condition is healed.*

In my own practice, I have used aloe vera only externally, although I know that some of the natives of the Pacific Islands and some Floridians take the jelly part of the plant internally for stomach ulcers and other digestive problems. A Hawaiian friend of mine swears by this method to cure or prevent stomach ulcers.

Again, let me emphasize that all these substances—zinc, vitamin E, and lecithin—are potent catalytic health vitalizers in their own right. Not only are they excellent to heal various skin conditions, but they also furnish the body with extra pep and energy when they are taken internally.

6

Preventing Infections and the Loss of Energy That Goes with Them with These Potent Catalytic Health Vitalizers

Although fruit and vegetable juices, those amazingly efficient catalytic health vitalizers I discussed in Chapter 1, furnish a great deal of the vitamins A and C so necessary to prevent or heal infections, sometimes a much larger amount is required to ward off an acute inflammation or to rebuild the body's tissues after a siege of sickness. It would be quite difficult to consume enough fruit and vegetable juices daily to yield the equivalent of 5 or 6,000 milligrams of vitamin C and 10 to 25 thousand units of vitamin A.

These two catalytic health vitalizers, vitamins A and C, are extremely important in maintaining high energy reserves when a person is healthy, or in restoring energy after an individual has been sick. Any infection, be it acute or chronic, no matter where it is located, depletes the body's energy. A hidden chronic infection is especially bothersome, for when a person's energy reserves are constantly being sapped, he drags around all day long, always feeling miserable, and never really knowing why. And acute infections can also be troublesome. You know quite well, I'm sure, how rotten and worn-out a simple cold or the flu can make you feel.

Vitamins A and C can do much to relieve the symptoms and solve those problems. If not enough A and C are in the diet, then the body's mucous membranes become especially susceptible to acute and chronic infections.

In the typical case histories I'll give you in this chapter, you will be able to see how ailments from asthma to urethritis were healed by the use of one of these wondrous catalytic health vitalizers. The first several examples deal with the use of vitamin A.

How Lester O's Severe Bronchial Asthma Was Relieved in Only One Short Week

About 6 months ago Lester had an acute attack of bronchial asthma. It was on a weekend and the only place professional treatment was available was in the local hospital's emergency room. Lester did not want to go there, but his asthma got so bad he could hardly breathe. In desperation, he called a friend who had an inhaler that he used for acute asthmatic attacks. This treatment gave Lester enough temporary relief to make it through Saturday afternoon and Sunday.

However, he was still very sick on Monday morning; so he made an appointment with his physician. The doctor gave Lester a shot of some sort and prescribed some medicine for him. Although the treatment did help Lester to breathe somewhat better, the medicine made him feel drowsy, dizzy, and so sick to his stomach that he was still unable to go to work that week.

Lester came to me on Friday to see if he could obtain some relief from natural healing methods. Knowing that vitamin A is usually deficient in the body in cases of asthma, I started Lester out at once on 50,000 international units of A each day, even before I completed my laboratory tests and dietary analysis. This is one huge advantage that natural healing methods have over drugs. I always know I will never hurt a patient with a vitamin, even if it isn't the exact one he needs. You can never say that about drugs.

As it turned out, vitamin A was exactly what Lester needed, and it was all he needed. In only one week, his symptoms disappeared completely. He was no longer short of breath, and, of course, with the vitamin A treatment, he suffered no side effects as he had with his previous medication.

I have since reduced Lester's vitamin A intake from 50,000 units a day down to 20,000. To experiment, we reduced it to 10,000 units a day once, which incidentally is twice the daily recommended allowance by the U.S. Food and Drug Administration, and Lester's symptoms of shortness of breath, wheezing, and coughing immediately returned.

Twenty-thousand units a day seem to be the minimum of this catalytic health energizer that Lester's body requires. As long as he takes this amount of vitamin A every day, he has no problem with his bronchial asthma, no matter how humid and warm the weather—and we have a lot of those days here in Florida—and regardless of how much he exerts himself.

This catalytic health energizer has not only restored Lester's ability to breathe without wheezing and coughing, but it has also increased his energy reserves. He does not fatigue as easily as he did before, and he says he has more drive and hustle than he used to.

How This Catalytic Health Vitalizer
Can Help You, Too

Although I do have 2 more case histories I want to tell you about in the use of vitamin A, I want to cover some other material about this catalytic health vitalizer first while Lester's case is still fresh in your mind.

There is always a great controversy as to what the daily

minimum requirements of vitamins and minerals are. This is about like trying to determine what the "minimum daily requirement" of the average person is for *water*.

I'm sure you can see immediately that the amount of water each person needs depends on how much salty food he has eaten, the temperature and humidity, his physical exertion, how big he is, how much he weighs, as well as various other factors. No 2 of us are ever exactly alike, either in our requirements for water or in our body's demands for vitamins and minerals.

In Lester's case, 4 times the minimum amount recommended as the correct daily allowance by the U.S. Food and Drug Administration was necessary to maintain his good health after he got well. Remember, though, at first when he was still sick, I had to use 50,000 units a day—10 times the FDA's recommendations—to relieve Lester's symptoms.

Nor did Lester have any bad side effects from this amount of vitamin A. I would like to set your mind at ease on this point right now, for some alarmists insist that a *great many* people "overdose" themselves dangerously with vitamins. This is simply not true. In all the history of medicine, there are only about 24 recorded cases of persons who took too much vitamin A and suffered any distress. *No fatalities have ever been reported.*

Signs and symptoms of vitamin A overdosage in these few recorded cases—sparse coarse hair, loss of hair in the eyebrows, a rough dry skin, and cracked lips—disappeared within 1 to 4 weeks after those people stopped their excessive consumption of vitamin A.

How much is too much, then? Well, *as an adult,* you need not be at all concerned about taking too much vitamin A unless you take *more than 100,000 units a day for a long, long time.*

According to the 13th edition of the Merck Manual,* which is known in the medical profession as the "Physician's Prescription Bible," chronic poisoning in older children and adults usually develops *after doses above 100,000 international units a day have been taken for many months.*

---

*Merck, Sharp & Dohme Research Laboratories, Rahway, New Jersey, a Division of Merck & Company, Inc., 1977.

In Lester's case, the proper amount of vitamin A was all that was necessary to relieve his asthma and restore his good health. However, if you yourself have asthma, I would also recommend the following procedures:

1. *Eat lots of fresh fruits and fresh vegetables and drink their juices.*

2. *Get the proper vitamins and minerals in your diet.* In addition to vitamin A, vitamins C and E are usually needed. C helps to desensitize the body and reduce the allergic manifestations of asthma. E helps to increase the oxygen supply to the body and helps the tissue cells use it more efficiently. I have also found calcium and magnesium to be helpful in asthma cases.

3. *Eliminate all refined white sugar and products containing it from your diet.* White sugar is an empty food. It supplies the body with nothing but calories and is responsible for a great many physical problems, especially digestive disturbances. Honey can be used as a natural sweetener. Honey itself is also valuable in treating both asthma and hay fever.

4. *Avoid packaged and processed man-made foods as much as possible.* A good rule of thumb to follow here is to *eat food that is born—not made.*

How I Got Rid of Maxine T's Constant Winter Colds and Flu with This Natural Health Vitalizer

Maxine had been plagued every winter with colds and the flu. She was always in a weakened condition and was constantly worn-out from lack of sleep due to her coughing at night. Every time she caught a cold, she lost her appetite and could not eat properly which further sapped her strength. She had reached the point where she caught a cold in November and never got rid of it until the next April. I saw her in the drugstore one day in late November buying some cough medicine and I said, "Maxine, why

97

don't you come to see me? I'll get rid of that cough for you for good."

When Maxine came the next day, I automatically assumed that 5 or 6,000 milligrams of vitamin C every day would solve her problem. After all, I have usually found vitamin C to be of great benefit in the prevention of colds and the flu or in cutting their duration short. I'm sure you, too, have either read about the value of heavy dosages of vitamin C to combat the common cold, or you may have already used it successfully yourself.

But I soon found out that in Maxine's case vitamin C was not the total answer. She was also highly deficient in vitamin A. Now, 2 of the most potent sources of vitamin A are liver and fish, neither of which Maxine liked or ate. So I placed her on 25,000 units of vitamin A immediately. That was in late November. She was over that cold by the first part of December, and then went through the entire winter without ever catching a cold again or coming down with the flu. Maxine had never experienced such freedom in the winter before from colds and the flu. She was absolutely astounded at the results she had gained from the consumption of vitamin A.

That was many years ago in Missouri where winters can be miserable. Maxine still lives in St. Louis. I have since moved to Florida to escape the cold weather. But I still hear from her every year at Christmas time. A little note scribbled at the bottom of her card says she still takes her vitamin A every day and has not had even the slightest sign of a cold for many years now.

Why This Catalytic Health Vitalizer
Can Prevent Colds and the Flu
for You, Too

Although vitamin C is extremely worthwhile for fighting that cold of yours, vitamin A is valuable to keep it from getting a foothold in the first place. Vitamin A is of particular importance in maintaining the integrity of the mucous membrances in the respiratory passages. Well-functioning cells here can, by their mucus flow and cilia action (tiny hairs that brush away damaging materials), help protect the body against airborne cancer-producing particles, just as they help prevent bacteria and viruses from getting a foothold and thereby protect against infectious disease.

Vitamin A is one of the 2 vitamins most Americans do not get enough of; C is the other. So you can never make a mistake by taking supplemental vitamin A even if you feel you are in good health.

Professor Jean Mayer says not enough vitamin A in the diet is one of the main causes of blindness in America today. Studies conducted in Canada show that a high percentage of the people there do not get enough vitamin A either.

This Same Natural Healing Method Cures a Long Standing Infection for Martin S.

As I have indicated, vitamin A is ever so necessary to maintain the integrity of the mucous membranes to keep foreign bacteria and viruses from invading and causing infection in the body. It is also important for healthy skin, for it protects against epithelial deterioration.

If not enough vitamin A is present in the diet, acne and other pustular skin conditions develop. I have found that this marvelous catalytic health vitalizer can bo uced not only to prevent such ailments from developing, but also to heal those conditions after they have become established. Take Martin S., for example.

For several years, Martin had a constant skin infection on the left side of his head above the ear. It ran from the temple clear back to the lower part of his neck where the hairline disappeared. It was approximately 2 inches wide. That area was constantly in a state of infection with eruptions that ran all the way from reddish pimples to pus-filled vesicles that would break open and crust over.

Martin had used a number of antibiotics, penicillin, ampicillin, erthyromycin, and so on. His doctor had also tried sulfa ointments. These medications would reduce the infection slightly for a few days or so, but as soon as the effects of the medicines wore off, the condition would be just as bad as ever. Once, Martin had painted the area with merthiolate, but he took such a ribbing at work about looking like an Indian, he never tried that treatment again. He was at wit's end when he came to see me.

I used 2 substances to help Martin get rid of his problem permanently. First, I asked him to get some pine-tar soap and use it to shampoo his hair with every day until the infection was cleared up. He was to use no other kind of soap or shampoo of any sort on his hair. Second, I had him take 50,000 units of vitamin A every day.

The results were both swift and positive. In only 10 days, Martin's scalp infection was completely gone. There was no sign whatever left of it. At that time I asked Martin to reduce his vitamin A to 25,000 units a day and to continue that amount indefinitely. I also recommended that he keep on using pine-tar soap to wash his hair and scalp, but that he could do that every other day or so rather than daily. Martin has followed my advice and has never once had a recurrence of his problem in 3 years.

How You Can Help a Head and Scalp Condition Yourself

Since I have already discussed the merits of that marvelous catalytic health energizer, vitamin A, I will limit my remarks here primarily to pine-tar soap, and tell you how it helped me.

I had been recalled to active duty with the army for the Korean War in 1951 and had picked up a scalp condition similar to Martin's while I was in Korea.

The army doctors used every possible antibiotic, sulfa drug, and skin ointment they could think of to cure my condition, but nothing helped. In January, 1952, my division, the 24th Infantry, was taken out of Korea to be stationed in Japan. One day while shopping in the Post Exchange, I happened to spot some pine-tar soap, and I remembered that my mother had used it often when I was a child. I could recognize the distinctive odor immediately.

I used this soap to rid myself of my scalp infection and at the end of 3 months I was finally free of it. Had I used vitamin A along with it, I'm sure my condition would have healed much sooner, just as Martin's did.

Since that time I have always recommended pine-tar soap and vitamin A for patients with any sort of a scalp problem. The results have always been positive. I might add that in the last several years I have asked patients to add 30 milligrams of zinc gluconate daily, for zinc helps speed up the body's healing processes in any sort of a skin infection.

Pine-tar soap does not have any fancy smelling chemicals in it to sensitize and irritate your skin, so it can really be effective in healing irritations and inflammations. If you have any children with teen-age acne, I would recommend it for them, too, along with the vitamin A and zinc.

How Bob W. Got Rid of His Deep-Seated Glandular Infection and Gained Increased Energy at the Same Time

Some time ago, Bob developed some hard lumps in his groin area that were extremely sore and painful to the touch. He was also running a temperature of slightly over 100, and he felt extremely tired and worn-out. Bob was afraid of cancer, as so many people are—and rightfully so, when a lump appears under the skin anywhere. So he went immediately to see his family medical doctor. Bob was told that it was nothing that serious, but that he did have a virus infection of some sort in the lymphatic glands.

The doctor gave Bob a penicillin shot and a prescription for oral penicillin for 10 days. He also told Bob to use moist warm compresses on the sore glands to relieve the pain and tenderness until the infection worked its way out.

Unfortunately, that did not happen altogether. The penicillin evidently kept the infection from spreading, for Bob's fever went down, but the lumps remained. They were still extremely painful, and they made it difficult for Bob to walk. Not only that, but he still was tired and worn-out and had no energy to do his job.

When he came home after work, he would drop in his easy chair immediately after eating supper and fall asleep. All this indicated that even though Bob no longer was running a temperature his infection was still present in his body.

For deep-seated infections, I have always found that the best catalytic health vitalizer to use is vitamin C. I asked Bob to start with 5,000 milligrams daily. In only a week the hard lumps had become softer and were diminishing in size. In 2 weeks they had completely disappeared along with the pain and tenderness.

The quick results really surprised Bob, but what amazed him even more was that vitamin C restored his energy levels. He no longer had that tired and worn-out feeling. He had plenty of zip throughout the day to do his job and instead of flopping down in the chair and going to sleep after supper, he was in his den working on his favorite hobby—antique guns.

How This Magnificent Catalytic Health Vitalizer Can Help You Cure an Infection

A great deal of information has been published in recent years about the value of vitamin C in fighting the common cold. Even television and movie stars have joined the ranks of those who support the "vitamin C movement to fight the common cold." Merv Griffin, for example, tells his audiences that he takes 2,500 milligrams of vitamin C daily and he has not had a cold for many years.

But very little attention has been paid to the ability of vitamin C to fight infections deep inside the body. Nor has much been said about how the deficiency of vitamin C can also lead to general debility and weakness and thus increase a person's susceptibility to infections.

It matters not where the infection is in the body; vitamin C can be of great assistance. Dr. Fred Klenner of Reidsville, North Carolina, has been a pioneer in the use of this potent catalytic health vitalizer to fight infections and inflammations. He uses vitamin C both orally and by injection with his patients. He says it is useful against bacterial and viral invasions of the body.

He has also obtained excellent results within 24 hours in

cases of monoxide poisoning and barbiturate poisoning. He has even used it successfully to heal a man who had been bitten by an extremely poisonous puss caterpillar. Dr. Klenner injected 12,000 milligrams of ascorbic acid directly into the bloodstream to neutralize the poison. Dr. Klenner says that except for the vitamin C, this man would have died from shock and asphyxiation.

In another case, a 4 year old girl was bitten on the leg by a poisonous snake. When she was brought to Dr. Klenner's office, she was vomiting and crying with pain and fright. While Dr. Klenner waited for an antivenom skin test reaction to determine which anti-venom to use, he gave her an injection of 4,000 milligrams of vitamin C. Even before the antivenom was given to her, the child had stopped crying and vomiting. She was laughing and drinking a glass of orange juice. A second injection of vitamin C restored her to normal.

Vitamin C has important anti-stress properties. A deficiency of it leads to nervousness, lassitude, and weakness. One example of this anti-stress property is that soldiers under the extreme strain and tension of battle always have drastically reduced vitamin C reserves in their bodies. This anti-stress property is one reason vitamin C is such an excellent catalytic health vitalizer.

Remember that vitamin C is one of the 2 vitamins in which most Americans are deficient. So even if you are in apparently good health, you would be wise to take a vitamin C supplement every day.

How much should you take? This, also, is about like trying to determine how much water you should drink in a day's time. However, from experience in my practice with many patients over the years, I have found that the best rule of thumb to follow is to take just enough to create a tiny bit of diarrhea and then back off from that amount by 500 to 1,000 milligrams.

I usually start my patients with 3 to 5,000 milligrams to fight an infection depending upon their size, weight, age, and so on. Some of them will be able to consume that amount with no problem, and in fact, will be able to take even more. However, there will always be a few who cannot tolerate more than a couple of thousand milligrams without getting a touch of diarrhea. I personally take 5 to 6,000 milligrams every day, increasing it to 10 or 12,000 milligrams if I feel that a cold might be starting, with no problem whatever from any diarrhea.

Vince A. Makes a Fantastic Recovery from His Troublesome Urethritis

Five years ago Vince suddenly came down with an attack of acute non-specific urethritis that developed into a chronic condition. It was extremely painful for him to urinate, for the sensation was that of scalding pain when passing water. He had a slight yellowish discharge which indicated the presence of pus cells in his urinary tract. He also had a high fever in the acute stages that never returned quite to normal as his problem became chronic.

Vince's family doctor sent him to a urologist for treatment. However, this specialist was not successful in culturing a urine specimen to determine the most effective drug to use. He had Vince admitted to the hospital for several days so that more extensive laboratory tests could be run, but none of these pinned down the exact cause of the urethritis. After leaving the hospital, Vince returned to the urologist for treatment, but after 6 months of numerous drugs and even a cauterization, he was no better. He was, however, as he told me, nearly a thousand dollars poorer.

Vince came to me, not really believing, but only hoping that perhaps some drugless natural system of healing might help. In addition to Vince's painful urethritis, I found that he was extremely weak and nervous. The stress and strain of his painful problem had completely exhausted his body's vitamin C reserves.

I decided then to attack his chronic infection with granular vitamin C that can be dissolved in water. I asked Vince to drink a glass of boiled water with 1,000 milligrams of granular vitamin C dissolved in it every waking hour for the next 3 days, regardless of whether he got diarrhea from this amount or not. At the end of 3 days, he was to return to the office for further examination.

When Vince came back in, he told me that his urination was much better. He no longer had the scalding pain when he went to the bathroom. Even the sticky yellow discharge had disappeared.

However, he still had a temperature of 99.6; so I knew his infection was not completely cleared up yet. I had him cut down his vitamin C intake to 6,000 milligrams a day and asked him to come back in another week.

When Vince returned to the office this time, his temperature was down to normal. He had no symptoms whatever of his urethritis. His urine was clean and crystal clear. A subsequent microscopic examination of a urine specimen by a laboratory confirmed this finding.

And thanks to the catalytic energizing properties of vitamin C, Vince no longer felt dragged down and worn-out. His energy had been completely restored. Vince has continued to take 3,000 milligrams of vitamin C during the past 4 1/2 years and has never once had a single sign of his previous problem.

Joyce K. Quickly Gains Relief from Recurring Cystitis with This Astounding New Treatment

Joyce had suffered for many years with a chronic recurring cystitis. During the acute attacks, which would occur every other month or so, she had a deep pain in the lower abdomen that ran down the inner side of both thighs. She had a constant desire to urinate, even after just going to the bathroom. Her urine burned, and there were signs of both blood and pus during the acute phases.

Various doctors had prescribed every possible antibiotic, and these would help Joyce temporarily. But her body would then either become adjusted to the antibiotic or allergic to it; so it would have to be stopped.

After hundreds of dollars worth of x-rays, uncomfortable, time-consuming, and expensive laboratory tests and physical examination, along with untold amounts of nauseating antibiotics, Joyce gave up on the medical approach to her problem and came to me.

I immediately used the same treatment on Joyce that I had used with Vince: a glass of boiled water with 1,000 milligrams of granular vitamin C dissolved in it every waking hour for 3 days.

At the end of that time, I had her go to 6,000 milligrams a day.

After her acute symptoms of pain and scalding urine disappeared, which took about 3 weeks, I reduced her intake to 2,000 milligrams a day on a permanent basis. This amount has kept her free from her cystitis for more than 2 years now. Monthly checks of her urine show it to be clean, clear, and free of any pus, blood, or bacteria.

How You Can Rid Yourself of a Deep-Seated Chronic Infection

If you have been troubled with a deep-seated infection in your body that has not responded to antibiotics, then this catalytic health vitalizer—vitamin C—could well be the answer to your problem. Vitamin C is nature's way of curing an infection.

When that infection is healed, I know your energy reserves will also rise. Infections of any sort drag a person down; so you can't help but have more zip and pep when the infection is gone.

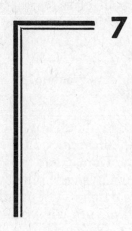 **7**

Putting a Magnificent Health Invigorator to Work in Your Body

The particular catalytic health vitalizer you'll read about in this chapter is one of the most potent you can find; it will increase your energy tremendously. It also protects and nourishes your entire nervous system. For instance, certain cardiac conditions have responded to its use, for the nerves affecting the heart need it for smooth, quiet, and effortless function.

This magnificent health invigorator contains essential nutrients for all the endocrine glands regulating the internal functions of your body. It aids in the formation of red blood cells, another energy booster. This catalytic health vitalizer is definitely an "upper," but without the bad side effects of drugs.

So if you are tired and irritable, if you feel you need a tranquilizer to calm your nerves, if you suffer from poor digestion, constipation, insomnia, neuritis, or anemia, then this catalytic health vitalizer could do wonders for you.

I have used it successfully for a variety of ailments, including the ones I have just mentioned, as well as Ménière's Syndrome, menstrual problems, edema, migraine headaches, and loss of memory. Let me cover a few of these case histories so you can see for yourself how well this magnificent health invigorator could work for you.

How Jane D. Solved Her Severe Loss of Memory Problem with This Amazing Catalytic Health Vitalizer

I had read in my nutritional science textbook how a certain factor of the vitamin B complex, *pantothenic acid,* could restore one's memory, but until I received a letter from a reader of one of my books, Ms. Jane D., I had never known of a case personally. I have covered Jane's case history in more detail than I usually do, for I found her story to be fascinating. I'm sure you will, too.

Jane is an executive secretary. She went back to work about 6 months ago for the same law firm that had released her the year before for inefficiency resulting from her unexplained loss of memory.

As Jane said in her letter, she couldn't even remember what day of the week it was. She was so mixed up that she often got dressed and went to work on Sunday only to find the office locked and no one there. Then she would forget to go to work on Monday until someone called to see if she was sick.

Or she would go to work in the morning, take off for lunch, and forget to return to the office in the afternoon. At home, she would sometimes forget that she had eaten supper and cook a full meal all over again at 11 o'clock at night. She said it was absolutely unbelievable the way she forgot things.

In the office, she'd be using shorthand to take down what her boss dictated and completely forget what he said right in the middle of the sentence. She got so bad that she couldn't remember her shorthand, and she'd been using it for more than 20 years. Often, she would fail to tell her boss when important phone calls came for him. Or people would come to see him and give Jane their names, and she couldn't remember who they were by the time she got her boss on the intercom. Sometimes, she wouldn't know why she had buzzed after she got him. On occasion, she couldn't even recall the office telephone number and the street address.

Jane went to medical doctors, several neurologists, and one psychiatrist. None of them helped her for they had absolutely no idea what was wrong with her. She even had a brain scan to see if she had a tumor, but that was negative. Finally, her boss had to let her go, although with great reluctance, for Jane was a highly skilled legal secretary. As Jane said, "He really had no other choice, even though he hated to do so."

After she was let go, Jane moped around her apartment for a while feeling sorry for herself. She was bitter and couldn't understand what had happened to her, for she had been a straight A student in both high school and college as well as an efficient legal secretary for more than 20 years.

Jane knew she wasn't mentally deficient and wondered if her loss of memory might possibly be stemming from a nutritional insufficiency of some sort. So she made one last visit to see a doctor, but as she said, he almost laughed in her face when she suggested that. She has never been back to see a doctor since then.

Jane decided to find out what was wrong for herself. She did a lot of reading about the human body—physiology, nutrition, and diet. She read some books on vitamins, minerals, and natural foods, and subscribed to several health magazines. She also began taking a multi-vitamin, multi-mineral supplement. Although this helped her general health, it did not improve her memory at all.

Then one day she read about a man who had taken pantothenic acid and found it suddenly improved his memory. She decided to try it. She got some 100 milligram tablets and started taking one with each meal along with her other multi-vitamin supplement. And then the miracle happened. As Jane said, "Wonder of wonders! I suddenly found I could remember everything again clearly and distinctly. My memory problem vanished into thin air. But of course I still didn't have my old job back yet."

Jane went to see her old boss, but he wasn't convinced. He just couldn't see how a vitamin could restore Jane's memory. Jane told him she didn't understand either, but she didn't care how it worked. All she knew was that she was now well and had her memory back again.

After a long discussion, Jane's boss told her he would consider taking her back if she could pass a certain test. They would go see a movie, and after it was over, if Jane could tell him all about it in full detail, he would take her back on a 30 day trial period. That's the most he would promise her.

Well, they did just that. They went to a see a long, complicated, and intricately plotted movie with an extremely large cast of characters. Afterward, Jane was able to tell her boss in complete detail everything that had happened. She even described fully the clothes the actors and actresses had worn, the scenery, the dialogue, and many points that he had overlooked or completely forgotten.

So Jane's boss took her back on a 30 day trial period after that movie. That was 6 months ago. She has no further problem with her memory loss as long as she takes 300 milligrams of pantothenic acid each day.

Another Fantastic Case of Memory Recovery

I have had one case in my practice similar to Jane's. Helen B. came to see me for her loss of memory problem, fortunately, after I had received Jane's letter. She, too, like Jane, had been to several doctors, a neurological clinic, and a psychiatrist, but had received no help whatever.

When I examined Helen, I found her intake of the vitamin B complex to be extremely deficient. Since I now knew and had some documented proof that pantothenic acid could help loss of memory, I had Helen take a 100 milligram tablet with each meal and one before going to bed, for a total of 400 milligrams a day.

I also gave Helen a complete B complex supplement along with some brewer's yeast and desiccated liver for good measure, for it is always wise to take the entire B complex rather than just one of the B vitamins by itself. The whole complex is necessary to get the best results even when a person seems to be deficient in only one of the individual B vitamins.

Has pantothenic acid helped Helen? You can judge for yourself, for here's what she says: "Since I began taking pantothenic acid, I can remember what I went into the next room for. I know what day of the week it is. I can remember where I'm going when I get in the car and start driving. I can even recall what I want at the supermarket without making up a long written grocery list. It's really a wonderful feeling of relief to know I'm not losing my mind and that all I needed was some pantothenic acid."

These 2 case histories may sound far-fetched to someone unfamiliar with the marked benefits that can be obtained through the use of such catalytic health vitalizers as vitamins, minerals, and natural foods. But they are not far-fetched at all. Scientific evidence has now shown that pantothenic acid can help people who suffer from *Korsakoff's syndrome*, a disease marked by loss of memory for recent events. The patient is disoriented, especially in reference to time. Korsakoff's syndrome is treated with large amounts of pantothenic acid along with the rest of the B complex for proper balance.

What You Can Do if You Suffer from Memory Loss Yourself

If you have problems with a failing memory, perhaps it isn't your fault after all. And it's just not because you're getting old either. You could need some more pantothenic acid. Or if Johnny and Sue bring home poor grades from school, the teacher tells you they just can't seem to learn, or they don't remember what you tell them. Try some pantothenic acid on them, too. Not only can it improve their memories, but it can improve your family relationships, too.

111

And who knows, if you have gray hair, it might start turning dark again. That is a pleasant side effect I've seen in several cases of pantothenic acid supplementation in my own practice.

How This Wonderful Catalytic Health Vitalizer Overcame Ménière's Syndrome for Clark J.

Ménière's Syndrome is a disease of the inner ear of unknown origin, characterized by recurring attacks of deafness, ringing in the ears, dizziness, nausea, vomiting, and double vision. The person tends to fall to the side of the affected ear and often cannot walk without help.

When Clark J. came to my office, he was not only troubled with all these symptoms, but he also could not bend over without falling on the floor. He had come down with the disease 6 months before and had been unable to work at his job in an automobile assembly plant since then because of the danger of falling into the machinery and permanently injuring himself.

At times his nausea was so violent that he could not hold down fluids of any sort. As Clark told me, on those occasions he did not dare come to the dining table. He would try to take some orange juice at the kitchen sink, but as soon as it hit his stomach, back up it came. If he had to go to the bathroom during the night, the only way he could be sure of getting there without falling down and hurting himself was to crawl on his hands and knees.

Clark had been to several doctors who told him he could easily have this problem off and on for the rest of his life, for there was no known cure. The only medication offered was a drug called "antivert." This was supposed to help his nausea and dizziness, but it did nothing whatever for him.

I'd never been faced with a case of Ménière's Syndrome before; so I turned to my *Doctor's Handbook of Nutritional Science.* There I found several case histories of this disease that had been treated successfully by heavy intakes of the vitamin B complex.

An analysis of Clark's dietary habits indicated he was extremely deficient in the vitamin B complex, so we started immediately with megadoses of B, brewer's yeast, and desiccated liver 4 times a day.

Clark did not become well overnight, but he improved slowly and gradually until at the end of 2 months he was completely free of all his symptoms and had returned to work. That was more than 2 years ago. Clark has continued to take his vitamin B supplements each day, although at a reduced dosage, and has not had an attack during that time. He says he feels better and has more energy than he has had in years. The vitamin B complex has acted as a tremendous catalytic health energizer for Clark, not only curing his illness, but also giving him increased strength and vigor and an overall feeling of well-being.

Now you may never suffer with Ménière's Syndrome, but if you ever are troubled with dizziness or nausea at times, double vision or ringing in the ears, take some extra vitamin B. It could solve those problems for you quickly. I do know one thing for sure: vitamin B along with some brewer's yeast and desiccated liver can give you that extra shot of energy you're looking for to get through a tough day, no matter whether it's at the office or home with the kids.

How Marilynn P's Menstrual Problems Were Amazingly Eliminated

A lot of women suffer needlessly at the time of their menstrual periods and before. Unfortunately, too many of them accept their problem as being a normal female nuisance and do nothing about it. Marilynn was one such person until she finally became completely disgusted with the situation as it was and came to me to see if there could possibly be a nutritional solution to her problem.

As Marilynn told me, she became a veritable witch, especially during her premenstrual phase. Her abdomen would bloat and her breasts swelled up and became extremely tender, all due to water storage. She would become quarrelsome, irritable, and depressed. In fact, she was so hard to live with that her children would avoid her and her husband would stay late at his office to keep from coming home.

I told Marilynn I had solved this problem for other women very quickly and simply by having them take megadoses of the vitamin B complex 4 times a day. In addition to the vitamin B, I asked Marilynn to eat often during her premenstrual periods (high protein foods, but not sweets), avoid drinking too much coffee since it disturbed blood sugar levels, and to take in more calcium in the form of dolomite to help settle her nerves and eliminate tension.

By following this simple but highly effective program, Marilynn found she was able to avoid her temporary premenstrual and menstrual discomforts. As she told me, she thought her husband and her children were even happier than she was now that her problem was solved.

How You Can Benefit from Marilynn's Case History

If you have been having menstrual problems such as Marilynn had, use some mega-dosages of the vitamin B complex. This marvelous catalytic health energizer helps maintain the proper sodium and potassium balance in the body. These 2 minerals are primarily responsible for the regulation of body fluids. Thus, the vitamin B complex helps get rid of the premenstrual edema without the use of diuretic drugs, which can so often cause serious side effects.

This ability of the vitamin B complex to eliminate excess water from the body can be helpful in many other ways, too. For instance, I have had some women patients, whose hands were so swollen they could not wear a ring or thread a needle, become completely normal again with the use of this potent catalytic health vitalizer. Let me give you an example of just one such case.

How Nina L's Problem Was Completely Solved Almost Overnight

Nina was almost frantic when she came to my office. Her feet and ankles were so swollen that it was extremely painful for her to walk. However, her main concern was her swollen hands and fingers. She earned her living as a stenotypist and also played a violin in a small city symphony orchestra. As she told me, her hands were her livelihood, and they were now so swollen and sore in the joints that she could barely function.

The vitamin B complex worked wonders for Nina. It drained off pounds of water. She no longer has any pain or soreness in her hands or feet and as she said, her fingers almost look skinny now.

Nina also noticed another wonderful benefit from this fabulous catalytic health vitalizer. Her spirits have been lifted tremendously; she feels much more alive and full of pep and energy. As Nina says, she almost feels as if she gets a "high" when she takes her vitamin B supplement.

Why Henry E. Was Able to Throw Away His "Water Pills"

When Henry was 62, he went into the hospital for elimination of excess body fluids that were causing a problem for him by placing an extra burden on his heart. Henry's feet and ankles were badly swollen and distended. They pitted distinctly with finger pressure. After 10 days in the hospital, during which time there were dozens of x-rays and several cardiograms, Henry was discharged with a prescription for 2 kinds of "water pills," and told to quit his job, go home, rest, and stay off his feet.

Henry had to quit his job as a real estate salesman and accept early social security retirement. He was now quite short of breath and could barely cross the street before he was winded. His chest would pain him severely at these times.

After a year of this, Henry was extremely despondent and

discouraged with life. He went to a prominent medical clinic in a nearby large city, but received no encouragement. The doctors there also prescribed complete rest, no work, and more water pills.

Completely depressed now, Henry went home again and resigned himself to his fate, as he put it. But one day a friend of his brought by a copy of *Prevention* magazine for Henry to read. It contained an article on the use of vitamin B for edema in pregnant women. This friend also gave Henry my name and telephone number and recommended to Henry that he call me. A few days later Henry did call for an appointment.

When I heard Henry's story, I immediately decided to put him on huge dosages of the vitamin B complex along with brewer's yeast and desiccated liver for good measure. Although I did not expect the vitamin B to cure Henry's heart problem, I knew that it would be helpful in reducing the edema in his feet and legs, and, therefore, would reduce the load on his heart.

And that is exactly what happened. Henry has been under my care for a year now. He has lost nearly 20 pounds, mostly water. He can now walk several miles on the level without becoming short of breath, but hills or steep grades still give him a bit of a problem. Henry is now working part time and is also very active in every other way. He feels he is in excellent health and notices that he has a lot more pep and energy than other men his age. Henry has no doubt but that this is due to the catalytic health energizer, vitamin B.

How You Can Get Rid of Excess Fluids Yourself

The vitamin B complex is the most reliable natural diuretic that I know of. A great many times, fluid retention is simply a result of improper sodium and potassium balance. The vitamin B complex helps to stabilize and restore the proper balance of these 2 minerals.

If fluid retention is a result of congestive heart failure (in this case the fluids concentrate in the feet and ankles and pit easily with finger pressure), vitamin B can still be of great value. I am not suggesting that the vitamin B complex will cure your heart problem. But I do know that it can reduce the load on your heart by getting rid of some of those excess fluids.

To correct your heart condition naturally, you may have to turn to vitamin E. (This is what I did for Henry—1,200 international units per day to strengthen his heart muscle.) I'll discuss this amazing catalytic health vitalizer and its use in chronic cardiac conditions completely in the next chapter.

How You Can Give Up Smoking with the Help of This Magnificent Health Vitalizer

If you've tried to stop smoking in the past and were unsuccessful, then the following information could be extremely useful to you.

Doctor Karen Inverness, a psychologist friend of mine, conducts a stop-smoking clinic. Karen says that up until 6 months ago, only about 30 percent of her clientele was able to quit smoking and make it stick. Since then, her success figures have jumped from 30 percent up to 70 percent. Here's what happened to make that drastic change.

Six months ago, a member of Alcoholics Anonymous told Karen how the vitamin B complex had helped his nervous tension when he stopped drinking. He said it helped him level out those deep valleys of doubt and depression, anger and frustration that he had to go through.

Karen passed this information on to her patients and found to her amazement that it really worked. She says when they have their group meetings now, she can tell who's on the "B Program" and who isn't by their attitudes and actions. Karen says the vitamin B complex is really helpful for some of the people who had tried to quit smoking before and failed have been able to stop now with the help of the vitamin B to calm their nerves.

If Karen's story will help only one of my readers stop smoking, then it has well earned its place in this book.

How This Catalytic Health Vitalizer Can Get Rid of Your Aches and Pains

One of the most powerful factors in the vitamin B complex is B-6 (pyridoxine). But most people do not get enough of it in their diets. Dr. John N. Ellis has found that pyridoxine is one of the most widespread vitamin deficiencies in the United States. Its absence in the diet causes many different kinds of muscle and nerve pains. According to Dr. Ellis, a pyridoxine deficiency may be directly related to rheumatism.

I have had patients with jumping pains—that is, pains that would be in the left arm one day and the right arm the next—respond extremely well to pyridoxine when all other therapeutic measures had failed.

If you happen to have muscle or nerve pains that appear and disappear in different parts of the body without rhyme or reason, try some pyridoxine yourself, say 300 to 600 milligrams per day. You could be pleasantly surprised. I know I've said it before, but I must repeat it here: Don't forget to take the entire B complex along with the pyridoxine for proper balance.

How to Put This Magnificent Health Invigorator to Work for You

I am sure you are by now wondering if you, too, can use this amazing catalytic health energizer to correct many of your own problems, or, better yet, to keep them from developing. The answer to that question is definitely "Yes."

The first question is, how much do you need? Part of that answer depends on how big you are. The bigger your body, the more cells you have and the greater your need for the vitamin B complex. Other factors also affect your vitamin B intake, for example: How much sugar do you use? How much alcohol do you drink? Does your diet consist primarily of man-made processed foods? If you consume a great deal of sugar, alcohol, and processed foods, your vitamin B demands will be high, not only because these items lack this amazing catalytic health vitalizer, but also because sugar and alcohol destroy the vitamin B complex in the body. Besides that, most man-made processed foods contain only 3 or 4 synthetic vitamins of the B complex, yet there are more than 20 B complex factors found in natural foods.

Foods rich in the vitamin B complex are liver, brewer's yeast, wheat germ, and blackstrap molasses. But if you are like most of us, you probably don't like many of those foods; so you would always be wise to take a vitamin B complex in the mega-dose size supplement.

Dr. Harold Rosenberg, M.D., past president of the International Academy of Preventive Medicine, recommends the following intake of the vitamin B complex for people of normal weight in the age bracket of 36 to 60 just for maintenance of good health. I have also shown the U.S. Food and Drug Administration's recommended daily allowance for comparison purposes.

	Ages 36–60: Normal Weight			FDA's Recommended Daily Allowance	
	Men	Women			
B-1 (Thiamin)	150–300	150–300	mg	1.5	mg
B-2 (Riboflavin)	50–100	50–100	mg	1.7	mg
B-3 (Niacin)	200–1,000	200–1,000	mg	20	mg
B-6 (Pyridoxine)	100–400	200–600	mg	2	mg
B-12	12–50	25–75	mcg	6	mcg
Biotin	0.3–0.6	0.3–0.6	mg	0.3	mg
Choline	250–1,000	250–1,000	mg	None given	
Folic Acid	2–5	2–5	mg	0.4	mg
Inositol	750–1,000	500–1,000	mg	None given	
PABA (Para-amino benzoic acid)	100	100	mg	None given	
Pantothenic Acid	100–200	100–200	mg	10	mg

mg = milligrams; mcg = micrograms

119

As you can see, the dosage recommended by Dr. Rosenberg just for maintenance of one's good health, not for the cure of any specific disease, is in some cases 300 times as much as the FDA's recommended daily allowance. You can get vitamin B capsules in the mega-dose size from your local health food store, or from many of the companies who advertise in *Prevention* magazine.

As I've already shown you, a great many factors affect how much of the vitamin B complex you need to correct your own individual ailment. The best answer as to how much you should take is that you ought to take enough to get the job done. This will require some experimentation on your part. The correct amount will give you a feeling of strength, vigor, and superior functioning of your body's systems.

You cannot overdose with this marvelous catalytic health vitalizer as you can with nerve pills, tranquilizers, or drugs. It is water soluble, and any excess leaves the body in the urine. That is one of the main reasons it is so important to take this magnificent health invigorator every day in a supplement form, for it cannot be stored in the body for future use.

8

How You Can Rapidly Resolve Circulatory and Cardiac Problems

One of the main requirements for abundant energy, especially in your heart and circulatory system, is an ample supply of oxygen. Whatever you can do to increase your intake of oxygen and speed up the elimination of carbon dioxide will help build up your energy.

First of all, you should know the effect of insufficient oxygen in your body. Whenever a cell is deprived of oxygen completely, it dies. In the case of cardiac tissue or brain cells, this happens very quickly. With other body cells it is a slower process. However, if the oxygen supply falls below a certain critical level, but not so low that the cell can no longer live, it will begin to function abnormally, and disease results.

What is the surest way of insuring an abundant supply of oxygen to all your tissue cells so none of this will happen? The surest way is taking an adequate daily supplement of the marvelous catalytic health vitalizer I'll tell you about in this chapter. When you do that, you'll not only be able to supply your body with abundant energy, but you'll also prevent or be able to heal such conditions as angina pectoris, coronary heart disease, intermittent claudication, phlebitis, atherosclerosis, among others.

How Glen O. Was Freed from His Wheelchair with This Phenomenal Treatment

Glen was 55 years old when I first saw him in my office. He had severe angina pectoris with extreme shortness of breath. Even too long a conversation would bring on an attack, causing excruciating pain in his upper chest that went up into the left side of his neck and then down the inside of his left arm. When this happened, Glen would often grab his left armpit. As he told me, it felt as if he'd been stabbed in the armpit with a sharp knife that was being twisted around. Glen had already suffered several coronary attacks and was using nitroglycerin medication. He could no longer walk and was confined to a wheelchair.

Since Glen's blood pressure was normal and he had no past history of a rheumatic heart ailment, I placed him on huge doses of vitamin E: 1,200 units 3 times a day for a total of 3,600 units daily. Within the month Glen's anginal pains had stopped. He has been free from his angina for more than 7 years now. He is no longer confined to a wheelchair; in fact, he gave that up only 3 months after he started his vitamin E treatment.

Glen now does a lot of hunting and fishing. He walks a couple of miles every day and plays 9 holes of golf twice a week. He also plays poker with some of his neighbors one night a week until one in the morning.

All in all, Glen leads a healthy, happy, and physically very active life for a man in his sixties. To tell the truth, he's a lot more energetic than a lot of men I know who are 10 years younger. When I see Glen today, full of energy the way he is, it's hard for me to realize that he came into my office as an invalid in a wheelchair just a few years ago.

Glen no longer takes 3,600 units of vitamin E each day. He is taking a maintenance dose of 1,200 units a day of this amazing catalytic health energizer that healed his heart and restored his health and vigorous zest for life.

How I Helped Alice H.
Make an Amazing Recovery from Angina

Five years ago Alice began having some severe pains that were very typical of angina. The pains began in the left side of her chest, went up into the left side of her arm, and then radiated down the inside of her left arm. These attacks would come several times a day, almost always after exertion of some sort, especially after a heavy meal. Anxiety would also precipitate these attacks. A physician diagnosed her problem as angina pectoris and prescribed nitroglycerin.

Alice tried to adjust her life style to a slower pace, and this did help somewhat, but she still had some bad attacks. She had heard from a friend that vitamin E was good for angina, and knowing that nitroglycerin would never cure her disease, she decided to try some vitamin E. However, she took only 30 units a day, the amount recommended by the U.S. Food and Drug Administration as the daily allowance for vitamin E. This gave her no relief whatever; so although she was reluctant to do so without a doctor's advice, she upped her intake to 100 units a day. Still, she gained no noticeable improvement.

At that time Alice came to me, for she did not want to further increase the amount she was taking on her own. Since she had no past history of rheumatic heart disease and her blood pressure was not too high (150 over 90), I immediately started her on 1,200 units a day.

Alice's improvement was immediate and fantastic. Her angina pains decreased, and the attacks became less frequent during her first week of treatment. Her last attack, an extremely mild one, occurred on the 8th day after she came to my office. She has never had one since then, and that is now more than 4 years ago.

Alice says she can now do whatever she wants to do physically without any problem at all. She is an avid bowler, participating in 2 leagues each week in the winter. She also bowls several games by herself almost every day. In the summer she spends a couple of hours each day in the swimming pool, "not lolling around," as she says, but actively swimming. Alice is now 59 years old. She feels that vitamin E saved her life. Alice says that the vitamin E not only gave her added energy, but it also made living well worthwhile again.

I especially wanted to include Alice's case history, for although it is not as dramatic a story as some that I have in my files, it does demonstrate vividly how important it is to take enough of this marvelous catalytic health vitalizer to get the job done.

How to Know if You Have Angina Pectoris

First of all, let me explain the pathology of angina pectoris. In this disease, the coronary arteries that bring blood to the heart are always on the borderline of insufficiency. This means that when a person is resting and there is no extra demand on the heart, there's just enough blood supply to keep it functioning.

However, any sudden extra demand on the heart—for instance, exercise, a heavy meal, anxiety, etc.—will bring on an attack, for then there is not enough blood with its fresh oxygen supply to enable the heart muscle to function properly.

The pain of an angina attack feels almost the same as the pain of a true coronary thrombosis. However, with rest, as soon as the extra demand on the heart is gone, the pain will pass without any actual blockage of any of the arteries of the heart.

During an angina attack, the person suffers with a gripping pain that usually starts in the upper chest, often in the left side, sometimes in the middle. This pain can go up into the neck and then down the inner side of the left arm. The word, *angina*, is Latin and means *suffocation*. This is how the patient will describe the attack. He feels as if he is actually going to smother to death.

124

The usual medical treatment for angina is a nitroglycerin tablet placed under the tongue when an attack starts. This helps ease the pain, and it can often give sudden dramatic relief. It is not a cure, however, for it does not solve the basic problem, which is not enough blood with its oxygen supply to the heart through the coronary arteries.

What You Can Do for Yourself if You Have Angina Pectoris

If you have angina, the best solution I know of is to use vitamin E, and here's why: Vitamin E helps increase the supply of oxygen to the heart, and it helps the heart use oxygen more efficiently. Since a lack of oxygen is the problem that triggers angina attacks, then the proper solution is to supply more oxygen to the heart by taking enough vitamin E to keep them from happening.

No other substance has ever been found that works as well as this marvelous catalytic health vitalizer in helping get the much needed oxygen to the heart. I have had patients who were once unable to even walk across the street without suffering anginal pain recover so completely with vitamin E that they can now climb several flights of stairs or walk a couple of miles without any trouble at all.

How much vitamin E should a person take? Enough to get the job done. I can specifically recall a patient whose angina was solved with only 400 units a day. Another, 800. Some needed as much as 2,400 or 3,600 units a day. On the average, most of my angina patients had their problems solved with 1,200 units a day.

Are there any precautions to be observed with the use of vitamin E? Yes, not only with angina, but also in the treatment of any heart problem. I discussed this previously on page 68, but it is important enough to repeat the information here.

If you take vitamin E for any reason whatever, do so judiciously if you have a past history of rheumatic heart disease or if you have high blood pressure. It is not that vitamin E is dangerous as so many drugs are; it is not. But it is so efficient in strengthening the heart muscle that if you do have high blood pressure, this stronger and firmer heart beat can cause your blood pressure to rise even higher for a short period of time.

If you've had rheumatic heart disease and part of your heart has been scarred and left weaker, causing a cardiac imbalance, vitamin E can improve the healthy part of the heart so dramatically that it can temporarily increase the imbalance even further.

If you have any doubts about your own case, consult a doctor who understands the value of vitamin E and who knows its capabilities in treating cardiovascular conditions. In my own practice, if a patient has a history of rheumatic heart disease or current high blood pressure, I will start with as little as 50 units a day, increasing this by 50 or 100 units each month, depending upon how the patient reacts, until the desired level is reached, all the while monitoring the blood pressure or the rheumatic heart carefully. This procedure, of course, quite naturally slows down the patient's recovery, but eventually his problem of angina or coronary disease can be resolved.

Two other points about vitamin E should be mentioned here. Do not take E and iron at the same time, for iron neutralizes the action of vitamin E. If you are taking iron in any form, take it at a different time of day than vitamin E. The other point is that mineral oil, which is used by some people to help constipation, dissolves vitamin E in the intestines and prevents its absorption into the body.

How Esther L. Miraculously Regained Her Good Health with This Extraordinary Catalytic Health Vitalizer

Esther developed a case of coronary artery thrombosis and was treated at a very famous east coast medical center. There she was put on a cholesterol free diet and given all sorts of medicines, including blood thinning drugs. None of this treatment was the least bit effective. When Esther left the center, she felt as if she had survived her heart attack not because of the treatment she had received, but in spite of it.

Esther's husband, Barney, brought her to me about a year

after she had suffered her heart attack. Esther could not even walk across the room without experiencing severe chest pains. She had been living the life of a semi-invalid ever since she left the center.

I put Esther on a vitamin E regimen at once—1,200 units a day—and within 7 days she began to feel better. She was no longer as short of breath, and she could walk around the house with very little pain in her chest. Within 6 weeks, she no longer knew that she ever had a heart problem. All her symptoms of cardiac thrombosis had completely disappeared.

I saw Esther again last summer when I made a trip to Arizona, where she and Barney now live. Esther looked wonderfully well. It was hard for us both to realize that nearly 20 years had passed since she had come to my office.

Esther is now in her seventies and has more energy than the average person in his fifties, all due to that fabulous catalytic health vitalizer, vitamin E, which she still takes every day. She swims daily in her own swimming pool and is an enthusiastic "rock hound," spending many hours climbing around the Arizona mountains looking for new specimens. I only hope I feel half as energetic and full of life as Esther does when I'm in my seventies.

How Paul G's Heart Was Restored After a Massive Coronary Attack

Paul G. was in the army and on field maneuvers in Europe when he suffered a massive heart attack. He was taken by ambulance to a field hospital, receiving oxygen treatment all the way. He was apparently dead on arrival, but one of the medical corpsmen had seen a slight flicker of one of Paul's eyelids and continued the oxygen even after the staff duty doctor said nothing more could be done. Amazingly, Paul began to breathe again and survived the attack. However, he was left a cardiac cripple and was discharged with full disability from the army.

He spent the next 2 years in and out of a VA hospital, and although he was seriously ill most of the time, he refused to remain in the hospital except during his most acute phases. He was forced to remain there once for 3 months when he suffered a second coronary occlusion. His treatment consisted of blood thinning medicines, a low cholesterol diet, and a drug of some sort that his doctor called a "high powered artery opener."

Paul spent his time either in bed or a wheelchair, for the slightest bit of exertion brought on pain in his chest and difficult breathing. After 3 years of this, his wife called me one day to see if I knew of anything that might ease Paul's condition. Neither she nor Paul had any hope of a complete recovery; they merely wanted some relief for him if that was possible.

Paul was too sick to come to the office; so I went to his home. Considering the length of time—nearly 6 years since he had suffered his first heart attack—I frankly held little hope for him, for although I had seen vitamin E perform some miraculous cures, I knew that even this marvelous catalytic health vitalizer had its limitations.

However, I started Paul on 800 units of vitamin E per day, raising it by 200 units each month until he was taking 1,600 units daily. Paul showed slow and gradual improvement after the first week of treatment and continued to improve until at the end of 6 months one would not recognize him as the same person.

A year after his vitamin E treatment began, Paul was completely recovered except, of course, for the scar tissue that remained in his heart from the coronary occlusions. He is more active than many men his age (55) and now owns his own business, a small printing shop, where he spends 10 to 12 hours a day, most of that up on his feet.

Paul plays 18 holes of golf every Thursday afternoon and swims each evening when he gets home from work. Unless the weather is too rainy, he jogs to and from his office each day, a round trip of 3 miles. I wonder how many of us "healthy" people are that active.

How This Amazing Catalytic Health Vitalizer Gave Wendell S. Back His Life

Wendell was extremely bitter after he suffered his heart attack. He was only 42 years old, and kept himself in the peak of physical condition, and had done everything possible to stay healthy.

He had never smoked and did not drink alcoholic beverages of any sort, not even beer. He watched his weight carefully, avoided foods rich in cholesterol, exercised every day, and made sure to get 8 hours sleep every night. He swam at least twice a week at the Y, and ran 2 miles every day no matter what the weather was like.

Wendell was the last person in the world you would expect to have a heart attack, but in spite of all his efforts he did suffer a coronary thrombosis and nearly died from it.

Wendell was my neighbor, and after he came home from the hospital, I visited him. He was very bitter and complained to me that he might as well have eaten everything he wanted to, drank, caroused around, and "raised hell" for all the good his "clean living" had done for him.

I explained to Wendell that no matter how well he followed all the advice on how to prevent a heart attack, all these precautions were useless if he did not have enought *anti-thrombin* (anti-blood-clotting agent) circulating in his blood vessels to prevent a coronary thrombosis and a resultant heart attack.

I also told Wendell that rather than sit around and gripe about his condition, he would be far better off to start vitamin E treatment now so the remaining good heart muscle would be strengthened and more oxygen made available to keep another heart attack from happening to him.

Since I was not Wendell's doctor, I advised him to check with his cardiologist about using vitamin E. This doctor did not think it would help, but he had no objection to its use, for he felt it would not hurt him. Wendell began with 800 units a day and built it up to 1,200 units daily over a period of 5 months.

At the end of that time he was so well that his physician took him off all medication, ran a cardiogram, and pronounced Wendell fit as a fiddle except for some small scar tissue left by the coronary occlusion. The doctor was especially surprised to see how small this scar tissue was.

Less than a year after his heart attack, Wendell resumed all his previous activities. He still watches his weight, does not smoke or drink, exercises daily, and gets 8 hours sleep every night. He has included, however, one more item in his program to prevent heart attacks, which is the most important one of all: 1,200 units of vitamin E every day.

How to Keep a Heart Attack from Happening to You

In a true heart attack where there is a sudden actual blockage or thrombosis of the coronary arteries—as opposed to the temporary insufficiency in the blood supply of angina pectoris—the person will have a sudden severe pain in the center of the chest, sometimes radiating across the chest into the neck and down the arms. The victim will feel a tight crushing sensation and experience a feeling of impending death. He will also suffer from shortness of breath.

One major difference between a coronary attack and angina is the severity of the symptoms. A second difference is that since a coronary artery has actually been blocked or occluded in coronary thrombosis, rest will not relieve the attack as in angina.

Immediate emergency treatment is imperative in almost every case of coronary thrombosis if the patient is to live. If the person does survive, several months will be needed for him to recuperate enough to return to a so-called normal life.

The main reason I included Wendell's case history was to show you that even though you use a variety of measures to prevent heart attack just as he did—not smoking or drinking, watching your weight, getting plenty of exercise, etc.—these by themselves are not enough.

The best insurance against a heart attack is to take vitamin E so you will have plenty of anti-thrombin circulating in your blood vessels.

Vitamin E is a natural anti-coagulant. When you have enough of it in your bloodstream, you will reduce the chances of having a blood clot forming that could block off your coronary arteries and stop the oxygen supply to your heart. Vitamin E also acts to dilate the blood vessels and open up new pathways in damaged circulation which will bypass clogged or hardened blood vessels.

What to Do if You've Already Had a Heart Attack

Ordinarily, heart attack victims have only one chance in 3 of living long enough to have any treatment at all. Sixty-five percent die suddenly or are dead on arrival at the hospital. Of those who survive, the fact is that with the treatment commonly used, a large number of them will have a second, and if they live through that, a third attack, and die at an early age.

Unfortunately, most of my heart patients come to me after the coronary has occurred rather than before. Yet, because of vitamin E's ability to act as an anti-coagulant, a clot dissolver, and a blood vessel dilator, the oxygen supply to the heart can be increased so the person is able to live a normal, active, and happy life again. Let me cover some of those features of vitamin E in more detail now.

Vitamin E decreases the heart's need for oxygen. It allows the heart muscle to use oxygen more efficiently. Its presence in the blood stream will prevent clotting in blood vessels and thus help prevent a second heart attack.

If vitamin E is given as soon as possible after the attack, it will minimize the extent of the damage to the heart by decreasing the affected area's need for oxygen. Also, by speeding up the opening of collateral circulation and by decreasing the oxygen need of the muscle around the affected area, it will support this zone and prevent any expansion of the thrombosis.

Vitamin E also prevents contraction of the scar tissue which replaces the area of heart muscle lost when the blood supply was cut off. Scar tissue contraction squeezes out blood vessels in the area involved and makes the condition worse. Vitamin E prevents that contraction.

Even if the patient is not fortunate enough to have vitamin E treatment immediately after the attack, results of megavitamin E therapy later on can still be of great value, as you have seen in the case histories I've shown you. If the scar tissue is large and already contracted, vitamin E will make the rest of the heart muscle function better due to the decrease of oxygen need. Collateral blood supply will be increased and the chances for clots in the major and minor blood vessels of the heart will be lessened. So vitamin E therapy helps the whole heart and the chances of a second or even a third heart attack are greatly reduced.

How long does it take for vitamin E to improve a damaged heart? No 2 people are alike, of course, but I have found that the first indication of response is seen in 7 to 10 days, and improvement will be fully developed in 2 to 4 months.

I have spent a great deal of time on angina pectoris and coronary occlusion or thrombosis, for heart attack is today the leading cause of death. I feel it is extremely important for you to be aware of the capabilities of vitamin E in the prevention of heart attack or in normalizing the heart as much as possible after an attack. This information could save your life.

Now, I do want to spend a few moments to tell you about some of the other things vitamin E can do. The first 3 case histories show how it can improve the circulation in the lower extremities.

Other Benefits That Can Be Gained by Using This Fantastic Health Vitalizer

1. *How Bill N. Completely Recovered from Intermittent Claudication.* Bill had trouble with his legs for 6 years. The disease was called intermittent claudication. This is a problem of poor circulation and causes pain, tension, and weakness after a person starts walking. The pain intensifies until walking becomes impossible. Bill had to stop work because of it. One month of 800 units a day of vitamin E cleared up the problem completely. He is now able to walk with no pain at all and has gone back to work again.

2. *Phlebitis Cured for Florence R. with Fabulous Results.* Florence suffered for many years with phlebitis which eventually broke down and formed an ulcer. This would heal for a while,

then break open again. After one severe bout of infection, she had to have surgery. By this time, a great deal of scar tissue had formed which would crack open and form more ulcers. Her doctor wanted to perform further surgery and a skin graft, but Florence refused and came to me.

I put her on 1,600 units of vitamin E each day and also used a vitamin E ointment externally. The results were like magic. The ulcers healed, the scar tissue became pliable, and there was no further skin breakage. The bulging veins flattened and became normal. Florence now takes 800 units a day. She still works, standing on her feet nearly 8 hours a day. I consider this an extremely tough test for vitamin E.

3. *Orville T. Gains Spectacular Results in Treatment of His Atherosclerosis.* About 6 years ago Orville suffered a severe bout with atherosclerosis. He would wake up around midnight with painful cramps in his right leg. He would walk the floor for half an hour to restore the circulation. The same thing happened again around 4 in the morning.

A doctor gave him capsules to ease the pain and pills to stimulate the circulation. The pain killing capsules worked, but the pills to increase the circulation did not. His doctor then told Orville the only solution was surgery and possibly amputation of the leg.

Orville came to me, for he refused such a drastic procedure. I gave him 1,600 units of vitamin E daily, and he gained complete relief in just a few months. He still takes 800 units a day and has had no more trouble for the past year.

4. *How Roy W. Increased His Energy in Extremely Short Order.* I especially wanted to include this case history, for it shows how vitamin E can do wonders to build up a person's energy and improve one's physical abilities.

Roy and I were playing golf in a foursome 6 months ago. We had to climb up a steep incline to reach the tee-off area on the 16th hole. When we reached the top, everyone was breathing hard except me, and I was the oldest in the group. When Roy asked me where I got all my energy, I simply replied, "From taking vitamin E."

133

The next day he was in my office to learn more about this marvelous catalytic health vitalizer. Roy had no ailment as such. He just wanted more energy; so I put him on 800 units of vitamin E per day. I was interested in the results, so I asked him to let me know at the end of a month how he felt. Here are the benefits he told me that he gained:

1. After only 2 weeks on vitamin E, he was able to think more clearly.

2. His reaction time was decreased. He was able to react more quickly to any situation, including driving. (This indicates the brain was getting more oxygen and was able to function better.)

3. He was no longer short of breath on the golf course or anywhere else.

4. He felt more relaxed and not as nervous and tense as before.

5. Roy said he could do a full day's work at the office without getting tired and still have enough energy to come home and work around the house or watch his favorite television program without falling asleep in the chair as he used to do.

9

The Secret of Overcoming the Fatigue Caused by Muscular Aches and Pains

The muscle and joint pains of arthritis, rheumatism, backache, and the like cause nervous strain along with muscular tension and contraction. All this causes exhaustion and fatigue. The classic example of how pain can cause tension that can then cause fatigue is the ordeal one goes through in the dentist's chair. Just the anticipation of the pain to come—even if it never does—causes a person to tense up and grip the arms of the dentist's chair until the knuckles turn white. When it's over, the patient almost crawls out of the chair, stiff and sore from the muscular, nervous, and mental strain, often more tired than if he had done a full day's

135

work. Whenever you have pain, no matter what the reason, the end result always looks like this:

Pain = nervous strain and muscular tension = fatigue

In this chapter I will give you several case histories that demonstrate a number of catalytic health vitalizers that can be used to solve this problem of muscular aches and pains and eliminate the exhaustion and fatigue that go with them.

**How Ralph P's Chronic Backache
Was Quickly Cured by This
Superb Catalytic Health Vitalizer**

Ralph is a driver of a big semi truck. He has a route from Tulsa, Oklahoma to St. Louis, Missouri, a long tough haul through a lot of rough country. The constant bouncing took its toll on Ralph's back until driving became absolute torture for him.

He tried everything he could think of to help: massage, heating pads, soft mattresses, hard mattresses, boards under the mattress, water beds, and so on, but nothing seemed to help. He still had his chronic nagging backache.

Ralph blamed it entirely on his occupation, for the pain in his lower back caused him to tighten up, and he found himself gripping the steering wheel so hard that the muscles in his arms and shoulders would become stiff and sore from the strain and tension. At the end of a trip, Ralph said he was so exhausted that he could hardly climb down out of the truck. His time off at the end of a round trip became a battle to work the soreness out of his muscles and get himself in shape for the next trip.

Although Ralph had been a driver for nearly 20 years, he was on the point of giving it up, pension and all, and finding a different job when he came to see me. A physical examination and x-ray of Ralph's lower back revealed no major problem. I next turned to his diet to see if I could discover something. A complete analysis showed him to be extremely deficient in vitamin C, which was not at all surprising to me. I have found a vitamin C deficiency to be present in nearly every case of low backache.

I placed Ralph on 3,000 milligrams of vitamin C daily. His response was immediate and dramatic. In less than 2 weeks, his backache completely disappeared. Ralph has continued this amount of vitamin C and his problem has never returned. The day before a trip he doubles his dosage to make sure Also, during the trip, if he notices his neck muscles or shoulders tightening up at all, he immediately takes another 1,000 milligrams right then and there. As long as he takes these precautions, he has no trouble. Except for the normal fatigue that accompanies any hard physical work, Ralph tells me he feels in the peak of condition at the end of a trip. Nor does he need the time to recuperate as he used to. Instead he uses it to enjoy some much needed relaxation and recreation with his family.

**How This Marvelous Catalytic
Health Vitalizer Can Help You, Too**

If you are plagued with a chronic backache yourself, as so many people are, take 3 or 4 thousand milligrams of vitamin C each day. You could be pleasantly surprised at the results.

I must admit that I do not know exactly why vitamin C helps relieve a backache; I only know that it does. It could be because it helps the body manufacture *collagen*, a binding glue-like substance that helps hold our bones and tissue cells together. At any rate, if you do have a chronic backache that has not been relieved by other measures, take some vitamin C for it. There'll be no dangerous side effects as there can be with certain highly advertised over-the-counter non-prescription drugs that claim to cure backache for you.

Two other points worth mentioning here are these: One, vitamin C is water-soluble and must be taken every day. It cannot be stored in the body as are A, D, and E, the oil-soluble vitamins. Second, any sort of nervous strain, tension, anxiety, or worry, as well as muscular activity, drastically increases the demand in your body for vitamin C. So the more nervous strain and tension you're faced with, the more vitamin C you will need, perhaps even as much as 8 or 10 thousand milligrams a day.

How This Catalytic Health Vitalizer
Solved Painful Leg Cramps
for Art E. and His Wife, Janice

Art and his wife, Janice, both in their early sixties, were an extremely active and life-loving couple. They played golf, bowled, swam, and belonged to a square dance club that met every other week for dinner and dancing from 9 PM until 1 in the morning.

The only problem both of them suffered with was cramping in the legs and feet. This was especially noticeable after their strenuous activity of square dancing. They had read that calcium often helps to solve this problem; so they started out with bonemeal. This they discarded for the more reliable dolomite and found they gained 50 to 60 percent relief. However, they were still troubled a great deal on the nights they went square dancing.

When they came to see me, I was somewhat puzzled as to how to proceed, for they were already taking vitamins C and E as well as calcium in the form of dolomite. A complete dietary analysis revealed little of consequence; so I sent some hair samples to a laboratory for a complete mineral analysis.

When the report came back, I felt sure we had isolated the problem, for the analysis indicated there was a definite deficiency in many of the trace minerals the body needs for proper functioning. This ticked my memory into gear, and I recalled that my wife had suffered cramps in the calves of her legs on her first pregnancy more than 30 years before. We had resolved the problem with *sea kelp*, the most reliable source of all the trace minerals we need.

So I put Art and Janice on sea kelp, and asked them to take 3 tablets a day for the first month, 2 a day for the second month, and 1 per day thereafter. The end results? Their leg cramps disappeared completely at the end of the first week, and they have had no sign of their problem for a full year now.

To play it safe, on dance nights, they take 3 tablets during the day to make sure no leg cramps will return. Art and Janice both

138

tell me sea kelp has not only solved this problem for them, but it has also given them a more restful night's sleep. They also say it has made them more alert and energetic and improved their sense of overall well-being.

How You Can Benefit from This Potent Catalytic Health Vitalizer

Sea kelp is one of the most reliable sources I know of for trace minerals. All the known minerals are found in sea kelp in almost direct proportion to the mineral content of your bloodstream. Seaweeds are able to convert inorganic elements into organic elements by the process of photosynthesis. Pure, unadulterated kelp, harvested from the sea, provides a rich source of such minerals as iodine, cobalt, manganese, iron, copper, sulphur, silicon, boron and zinc.

How can you know if you are deficient in some of these trace minerals? The best way is to have your doctor send a hair sample to a laboratory for analysis. One laboratory that does this kind of analysis is Parmae Laboratories, 7101 Carpenter Freeway, Dallas, Texas, 75235.

What kind of problems can a deficiency of trace minerals cause? For example, a shortage of iodine can cause listlessness and lack of energy, apathy and low blood pressure. Insufficient manganese can be responsible for back problems of all sorts as well as muscle fatigue and exhaustion. A lack of copper results in loss of hair or graying hair, skin rashes, and possible heart damage. Not enough zinc causes a low resistance to infection, slow healing, loss of sexual vigor and fertility, and psoriasis-like skin conditions. A shortage of chromium can result in diabetic-like symptoms.

To prevent these problems or to keep from having leg cramps like Art and Janice had, take sea kelp every day. Other ailments that have responded favorably to sea kelp, according to several prominent medical authorities, are high blood pressure, premature aging, allergies, constipation, rheumatism, and dropsy.

Doctors George L. Siefert and H. Curtis Wood, both of

Philadelphia, made a study of 400 pregnant women who had been placed on 3 kelp tablets daily. They found the blood count (hemoglobin) rose from 65 to 83 percent. They also found the following improvements took place:

1. Better color and quality of hair,
2. Less brittle fingernails,
3. Less bruising due to fragile capillaries,
4. Relief in certain kinds of skin problems,
5. Definite improvement in rheumatism and arthritis,
6. Relief in cases of such eye disturbances as iritis,
7. Less constipation,
8. Increased sense of well-being.

You could easily enjoy the same benefits with the use of 1 to 3 sea kelp tablets each day. You need observe only one precaution with its use. Some persons are sensitive to iodine; so if a skin rash should develop with sea kelp, discontinue its use at once and see your doctor. However, I have never seen this happen in my own practice, and over the years I have treated countless patients with sea kelp.

This Catalytic Health Vitalizer Cures Rheumatism for 63 Year Old Man

I mentioned this wonderful catalytic health vitalizer back in Chapter 7 on page 118 and told you that its absence could cause all sorts of muscular aches and pains, but I did not give you an example of its use. I want to do that right now.

I had used this catalytic health vitalizer before on numerous occasions to successfully treat rheumatic-like pains and stiffness, especially in the fingers and wrists; so when one particular patient did not respond to other therapeutic measures, I decided to use it on him, even though his arthritis was not in the hands.

Harlan B., a local county official, came to me complaining of arthritis pain in his ankles, knees, and lower spine. His ankles and knees were stiff and badly swollen. His knees were so bad he could not cross one leg over the other while sitting down. Walking or climbing stairs was so difficult for Harlan that he was afraid he would have to give up his job, for he was on the 3rd floor of the old county courthouse, and it had no elevators.

A dietary analysis had revealed that Harlan was deficient in both vitamin C and calcium. However, when he did not respond fully to this treatment, I decided to add the catalytic health vitalizer, pyridoxine (B-6), although I could find no evidence of a deficiency.

Harlan's response to pyridoxine was almost immediate. After he had taken 750 milligrams daily for 2 weeks, his pain and swelling subsided completely. "I thought I was going to have to retire," Harlan told me, "but now I can climb the stairs to my third floor office without any trouble at all."

Harlan has had no recurrence of his rheumatism for the past 2 years. He will soon be 65 and is going to retire then, not for reasons of ill health, but simply because of age. "I feel so good now I think I could go on for another 5 years or more," Harlan told me the other day, "but I want to have some time of my own now to spend with my grandchildren."

How You Can Use This Exceptional Catalytic Health Vitalizer Yourself

If you have painful rheumatism or arthritis that has not responded to other therapy, use some pyridoxine. You cannot take too much, for it is harmless. However, 750 to 800 milligrams per day should be sufficient. Don't forget to take the rest of the vitamin B complex along with it for proper balance.

A quick way to find out if you are deficient in pyridoxine is this: Extend your hand with the palm up and the wrist straight. Now bend the first 2 joints in your fingers until they reach your hand. Do not bend the knuckles that are between the back of the hand and your fingers as you would in making a fist. You should bend only the first 2 joints of each finger to touch your hand.

If you cannot bend your finger joints this way, if you cannot reach your hand with them without making a doubled-up fist, then chances are great you have a pyridoxine deficiency.

Pyridoxine has been used to treat a variety of other conditions. Some doctors have reported success with its use in hypoglycemia, neuritis, Parkinson's disease, Bell's palsy, edema, muscle spasms, gastritis, and colitis.

Why This Fantastic Health Vitalizer Is Invaluable in Treating Muscle Spasms

One of the best treatments for muscular aches and pains, tenderness and soreness, is the fantastic health vitalizer, calcium. Let me give you just a few quick examples:

1. *Sore and Aching Muscles.* Constance M. was continually troubled with sore and aching muscles in her arms and legs. She had tried any number of liniments and ointments, but she received only partial and temporary relief. I asked her to take 2,000 milligrams of calcium each day in the form of dolomite. Constance found this did the job for her. She was free of pain within the week and has remained that way as long as she takes her calcium daily.

Constance also gained an unlooked for but welcome fringe benefit from this invaluable catalytic health vitalizer. She had been troubled with constant headaches for longer than she could remember. The calcium gave her miraculous relief from them.

2. *Muscle Spasms.* Jerry C. was bothered by muscle spasms in his right arm. They started underneath his right shoulder blade and went down the muscle beneath his arm from the shoulder to the elbow. Muscle relaxant shots and drugs proved to be useless; he still had his problem. Even pain-killers were losing their effectiveness.

Jerry was a carpenter, and since he was right-handed, the muscle pain and spasms greatly interfered with his work.

I asked Jerry to take 3,000 milligrams of calcium each day, divided into 4 equal portions—750 milligrams at breakfast, dinner, supper, and before going to bed. I also asked him to carry some dolomite tablets in his pocket on the job and to take 2 or 3 if his arm started to bother him.

This remedy was so effective that Jerry could hardly believe it, especially in view of what he had been through trying to cure his ailment. He found himself to be completely free from pain in only a few days for the first time in 6 months. He has been taking dolomite for 3 months now and has had no return of his former problem.

3. *Muscle Pain, Soreness, and Stiffness.* Ada L. was troubled with pain, soreness, and stiffness in her right arm, especially in the elbow. She could not even lift a cup of coffee to her mouth without suffering extreme pain. Her doctor told her she had *tendonitis* and gave her some cortisone shots. However, these did not help; in fact, Ada said they made her sick.

I put Ada on 5,000 milligrams of calcium in the form of dolomite. The pain became less and less noticeable and at the end of a month it was completely gone. It has never returned for more than a year now. Ada no longer takes 5,000 milligrams of calcium, but she does take 2,000 milligrams daily to play it safe.

4. *Sore and Aching Feet.* Brenda F. had for years been plagued with sore and aching feet and painful muscles in the calves of both legs. She attributed this to her job in an electronics factory that required her to stand up most of the day. After work she would soak her feet in hot water and massage her legs for nearly an hour to relieve the pain and soreness. Brenda was also bothered by terrible cramps in her feet at night.

I asked her to take 4,000 milligrams of calcium each day for her problem. The results were absolutely fantastic. In only 2 weeks, Brenda's soreness and tenderness disappeared completely from her feet and legs. Nor has she had a sign of a cramp at night. She says she has much more energy than before and is not as tired at the end of the day as she used to be.

How You Can Enjoy the Benefits of This Wonderful Catalytic Health Vitalizer

Calcium is required for proper muscle relaxation. When you do not have enough calcium in your body, your muscles cannot relax and rest. They will be sore and tender, and you will often be troubled with "shooting pains" that jump all over the body without rhyme or reason. Calcium is also necessary for the nervous system to function properly. It will relieve muscular twitching and spasms effectively.

Calcium is also very useful as a painkiller, regardless of the source of the pain. Migraine headaches, which are so much trouble to many people, can often be relieved simply by taking calcium.

You need a liberal intake of calcium to steady your nerves, relax your muscles, relieve exhausting tension, restore your energy. I always give a patient at least 2,000 milligrams a day, sometimes as much as 5,000 milligrams a day in the case of an older person where calcium is often poorly absorbed.

I prefer dolomite to bone meal, for there is no possibility whatever of any danger due to an excess of dolomite. Bone meal contains phosphorus, and an excess of phosphorus can cause calcium losses in the urine. This is believed to be one cause of a calcium deficiency. Besides, phosphorus is well supplied in the average diet—perhaps too well, since it is present in meat, seafood, eggs, dairy products, and many vegetables. I have never once seen a patient who was deficient in his phosphorus intake; so I never use bone meal, only dolomite.

How a Different Catalytic Health Vitalizer Can Cure Leg Cramps

In the preceding chapter I discussed how vitamin E, one of the most amazing catalytic health vitalizers I have ever used, could relieve cardiovascular conditions including coronary thrombosis, angina pectoris, intermittent claudication, phlebitis, and atherosclerosis. At that time, I did not mention how useful it can be in treating muscular cramps in the legs and feet.

Leg and foot cramps are a definite indication of poor or impaired circulation. Cramps can often be the forerunner of far worse things to come. I have been able to relieve very quickly dozens and dozens of leg cramps with this marvelous catalytic health vitalizer. Let me give you a few quick examples.

OVERCOMING MUSCULAR ACHES AND PAINS

1. *Leg Cramps and Varicose Veins.* Stella D. suffered with leg cramps for 11 years. They were especially severe during her menstrual periods. At times the cramps were so painful she could not walk without limping. She was also troubled with varicose veins in her ankles.

I placed Stella on 1,200 units of vitamin E daily. In only 30 days her leg cramps were completely gone and she no longer had any bluish-purple discoloration in her ankles. Stella has continued to take 1,200 units of vitamin E every day for the past year and has had no recurrence of her problem.

2. *Another Case of Leg Cramps Solved.* One of Stella's neighbors had also been troubled with leg cramps. When she saw how quickly Stella's problem was solved, she immediately went to the health food store, bought some vitamin E capsules, and began treatment on her own. Stella said her friend took 1,200 units daily. In only a few days the leg cramps with which she had suffered for more than 4 years went away.

Luckily, Stella's friend had no history of rheumatic heart disease or high blood pressure. Otherwise, she could have had problems. To start with 1,200 units of vitamin E daily without knowing your physical condition is extremely unwise. Unless you are absolutely certain that you have no past history of rheumatic heart disease and unless you know that your blood pressure is normal for your age, you should not use this high a dosage of vitamin E in the beginning without a doctor's supervision. And even if you are sure, you would be far wiser to start with 1 or 2 hundred units daily and build up slowly by increasing that amount by 1 or 2 hundred units each month.

3. *Nocturnal Leg Cramps.* Howard L. suffered so badly with leg cramps at night that he wore heavy long winter underwear and heavy woolen socks to bed even in the hottest months in the summertime. This procedure helped reduce the severity of the cramps, but it did not stop them.

I asked Howard to start with 800 units of vitamin E each day. We built this up to 1,200 units daily in 2 months by increasing 200 units each month. The results? "A miracle!" Howard says.

He no longer wears any warm winter clothing to bed. In fact, he wears nothing on his legs, for his circulation has improved so much that he stays comfortably warm. He has had no sign of the leg cramps that troubled him previously.

Howard has also realized at least 2 fringe benefits from vitamin E, perhaps even more. His hair, which was completely silver when he began his treatment, is turning dark again. Also, Howard finds he has a far greater energy reserve than before, a valuable asset at any age, but extremely so when you're 85, as Howard is.

How You Can Improve Your Circulation

Cramps in the feet and legs are a sure sign of failing circulation in the lower extremities. It indicates that the body is not getting enough oxygen in that area to help remove the carbon dioxide and other waste products that cause the cramping and fatigue. Vitamin E not only strengthens the muscular walls in the blood vessels, but it also improves their elasticity so the blood is moved along faster. At the same time, vitamin E brings more oxygen to the area and helps the tissue cells use that oxygen more efficiently.

Vitamin E is the most reliable remedy I know of for nocturnal leg cramps, exercise cramps, the "restless leg syndrome"—in fact, any sort of muscular cramping.

Vitamin E is also useful in the treatment of varicose veins. You should not expect complete disappearance of a varicose vein, although that does occasionally happen. However, vitamin E does relieve the burden on the varicose vein by opening up alternate or collateral channels through which the blood can flow. It will relieve the aching and sense of heaviness most patients with varicose veins feel.

I have seen one case where vitamin E performed a literal miracle. My own son spent nearly 5 weeks in the hospital as a result of an auto accident. He was in intensive care for 5 days and was fed through the veins for 10 days. As a result, huge nodules developed in the veins of both arms. The surgeon said they would always be there.

However, when my son left the hospital, I placed him on

3,600 units of vitamin E daily, hoping to dissolve those knots of scar tissue. They completely disappeared in 6 months. Today there is no sign whatever of them, and his veins are perfectly smooth, flat, and normal, much to the amazement of the surgeon.

Rose's Terrible Knee Pains
Cured in Only One Day

Rose had twisted her knee badly when she stepped in a hole in the backyard and fell. The pain from the torn ligaments was so excruciating that the aspirin and codeine the doctor gave her were completely ineffective. She could get only 2 or 3 hours sleep a night, and after 5 nights of this she came to see me.

I placed her on both calcium and vitamin E and she slept that night for 8 hours completely pain-free for the first time since her fall.

Rose's case is an example of how more than one catalytic health energizer can be used to heal an ailment. Some doctors do not like combining treatments this way, feeling they do not know which one was responsible for healing the patient. I do not feel this way. I am not conducting a laboratory experiment. I am interested only in getting a sick patient well.

So today, I treat all cases of muscular aches and pains with a combination of 4 catalytic health vitalizers: *Calcium* in the form of dolomite, vitamins *C* and *E* and *trace minerals* in the form of sea kelp. I have been most happy with the results I have obtained.

If you suffer from this problem of muscular aches and pains or leg cramps, then use these 4 catalytic health vitalizers yourself. I know you'll be happy with the benefits you gain.

10

How You Can Rid Yourself of Insomnia and Increase Your "Go-Power" with Catalytic Vitalizing Action

Insomnia is one of the major causes of lack of energy. If you do not get the proper amount of sleep and rest, you cannot possibly be at your best the next day. Some of the major reasons for the inability to sleep are these:

1. *Pain or Discomfort of Any Kind.* Many health problems that are not as noticeable in the daytime can become extremely troublesome at night. For instance, sinusitis, nasal congestion, bronchitis, asthma, or any respiratory problem is always much worse at night. So is itching. A woman's menstrual cramps are also much more painful at night when she is lying down.

149

2. *Circulatory Diseases.* The "restless leg syndrome" or a circulatory disorder such as *Buerger's disease* or *acroparesthesia* can cause insomnia. In this situation, the primary disease causes the secondary problem of insomnia. I'll give you some case histories from my files to show you how these circulatory ailments can be healed. Then, of course, the insomnia is cured, too.

3. *Specific Nutritional Deficiencies.* The lack of certain catalytic health vitalizers, which I will discuss later on in this chapter, will cause insomnia. This problem can readily be corrected by the addition of the missing or partially deficient catalyzer.

4. *Insomnia Caused by Stimulants.* Coffee and tea are the 2 stimulants that always come to mind for most people. However, I think you'll be greatly surprised to find that an ordinary household condiment is by far the worst offender.

5. *Fear, Anxiety, and Worry.* Sometimes, the causes of insomnia are mental or emotional rather than physical. For instance, financial worries, marital problems, fear of failure—stress of any sort—can cause insomnia. Although I cannot resolve your specific problems individually for you in this area, I can give you some techniques and guidelines I have found to be most helpful for my patients.

Insomnia Caused by Pain or Discomfort of Any Sort

Pain of the spine or nerves can be especially troublesome at night. So can tension or migraine headaches. An upset stomach, no matter whether due to simple indigestion or some serious disease in the digestive tract, often wakes a person up out of a sound sleep.

Stomach ulcers are almost as dependable as an alarm clock. Unfortunately, they usually wake the person at 2 AM rather than 6 or 7. If you are being awakened regularly at this time with stomach pain every night, chances are you have a stomach ulcer. When that is healed, your insomnia will vanish, for it is only a secondary problem resulting from the primary condition.

Since I could not possibly cover all the conditions that cause pain or discomfort, and thus insomnia, in this chapter, I would recommend that you locate the remedy for your specific ailment elsewhere in this book, or in a previous book of mine, *Extraordinary Healing Secrets from a Doctor's Private Files.** This book contains a great deal of valuable information about home remedies for pain and discomfort. This book of remedies is available from the publisher, or it can be ordered through your bookstore.

Insomnia Caused
by Circulatory Diseases

MORGAN C'S INSOMNIA DISAPPEARS
WHEN HIS BUERGER'S DISEASE IS GONE

Several years ago, Morgan began having trouble with his right leg. The foot and calf became quite painful when he walked. In fact, he could go no more than 2 blocks before the severity of the pain would cause him to stop. His foot was cold most of the time.

At night, Morgan would have to get out of bed every couple of hours and walk about for 15 minutes to get the circulation going and relieve the pain. The only way he could sleep at all was to let his foot hang out over the edge of his bed.

His doctor at that time diagnosed his problem as *Buerger's disease*, an ailment where the patient suffers from an inflammation of the inner walls of small blood vessels along with constriction and clogging because of blood clots. The doctor told Morgan his condition was incurable since there was no known specific medical therapy for Buerger's disease.

So when Morgan came to see me, he did not come to get help for Buerger's disease, for he thought nothing could be done for that. He came to see if I could do something for his insomnia. However, as I told Morgan, something could be done to help his

---

*James K. Van Fleet, *Extraordinary Healing Secrets from a Doctor's Private Files* (West Nyack, New York, 10994: Parker Publishing Co.), 1977.

circulatory problem. When that was solved, then his insomnia would automatically disappear.

And that's exactly how it happened. I immediately put Morgan on 2,400 units of vitamin E daily. The first sign of improvement was a decrease in the pain. Then his foot lost the bluish-purple color it had been when he came to the office. It also became warmer, indicating that the circulation was better. In only 6 short weeks, Morgan was completely weil and his insomnia was also gone.

Morgan has been under my care for nearly a year now. There has been no sign of his previous circulatory problem. He has no pain in his foot or leg, no matter how far he walks. He sleeps all night without waking up. His energy seems unlimited. As Morgan says, he never seems to tire out. We have reduced the amount of vitamin E he took in the beginning, but he still takes 1,200 units each day.

HOW THIS CATALYTIC HEALTH VITALIZER
CURED KEITH Y'S "RESTLESS LEG SYNDROME"

The "restless leg syndrome" is a circulatory condition that affects middle-aged men about 10 times as often as it does women. The problem is more noticeable at night. The person's legs twitch and jerk with nervous and muscular spasms.

Keith's problem was so bad that he would wake up out of a sound sleep with his legs jerking. Then he would be unable to go back to sleep again. In the morning, instead of being rested and ready to go, he was exhausted.

I immediately placed Keith on 1,600 units of vitamin E, and his restless leg syndrome disappeared in less than a week. He was no longer nervous and jumpy in the daytime, and he was not awakened any more during the night. His wife called to thank me, for Keith was no longer short-tempered and grouchy, as he had been before when he was troubled with this condition.

ACROPARESTHESIA SOLVED QUICKLY BY THIS
AMAZING CATALYTIC HEALTH VITALIZER

About 5 years ago, when he was only 59, Adam S. came to see me because he was unable to get a decent night's sleep. His arms and legs constantly became numb and went to sleep on him. His condition became so painful that he would wake up half a dozen times a night. Adam's doctor at that time told him he had *acroparesthesia*, a long-winded medical term that describes the tingling numbness a person feels when his hand or foot goes to sleep. The doctor said it was due to poor circulation because of Adam's age, and he said nothing could be done for him. He did prescribe some sleeping pills for Adam, but that was all he could offer.

My examination of Adam indicated that he had a circulatory ailment. However, I did not consider his condition incurable as his previous doctor had. I placed him on 1,600 units of vitamin E at once since he did not have a high blood pressure problem and he had never had a rheumatic heart condition.

Adam responded magnificently to the vitamin E treatment. In only 2 weeks, his problem was solved. His arms and legs no longer went to sleep on him. And his energy reserves were much higher than before, thanks to the catalytic health energizer, vitamin E. As Adam himself says, "I sleep like a baby, Doc. Don't know what it is to have insomnia anymore. Feel like a million, thanks to you!"

WHAT TO DO IF YOU HAVE CIRCULATORY PROBLEMS THAT CAUSE INSOMNIA

If you are troubled with any of these circulatory problems that keep you awake at night—for instance, Buerger's disease, restless leg syndrome, acroparesthesia, or nocturnal leg cramps —then take 1,200 to 1,600 units of vitamin E each day. You should see improvement within 2 to 6 weeks. Just be sure to observe the precautions I have mentioned before about vitamin E usage (high blood pressure or a history of rheumatic heart disease).

If you have Buerger's disease or any ailment that slows down circulation in your feet and legs, I would recommend that you not smoke. Cigarettes will only make the condition worse by constricting the blood vessels even further.

If you are bothered by the restless leg syndrome, and it does not respond completely to vitamin E therapy alone, then I would suggest that you also take 2,000 milligrams of calcium each day in the form of dolomite along with the vitamin E.

Calcium can be extremely helpful in nervous and muscular conditions. In fact, if, in addition to the jumping and twitching legs at night, you find yourself tapping your fingers, swinging your crossed leg or jumping at the slightest noise, or if you cannot stand sitting in one place for very long, there is no doubt about it—you need calcium as well as vitamin E. These 2 catalytic health energizers together will calm your nerves, give you a better disposition, and assure you of a good night's sleep, naturally, without sleeping pills or nerve tranquilizers.

Insomnia Caused by Stimulants

Certain foods or drinks are supposed to cause insomnia. The 2 most often blamed are coffee and tea. Yet I've known people who could drink several cups of coffee before going to bed and still go right to sleep.

I have long felt that it isn't the coffee or tea that keeps a person awake, but the liquid that is causing pressure on the bladder. If coffee or tea keeps you awake, I would bet that milk or water will do the same.

I have tested this on myself many times. If I drink 2 or 3 cups of coffee or tea or 2 or 3 cups of water or milk before going to bed, I will stay awake with the water or milk just as much as I will with the coffee or tea. As soon as my bladder is finally emptied, I will go to sleep at once, no matter which one I drank.

Of course, if you do think that coffee or tea will keep you from sleeping, I can assure you that it will. This is the classic example of mind over matter. For instance, in one study of sleep and insomnia, the caffeine was removed from the coffee and put into hot milk. All the patients who unknowingly received the caffeine in the milk slept peacefully. But those who drank the coffee without knowing it was decaffeinated did not sleep at all.

Although ordinary table salt is not usually thought of as a stimulant, it is. A French doctor, Professor Coirault, found that he could cure a patient's insomnia simply by cutting down on his salt intake. The professor says that sodium and potassium are natural enemies in the body's chemistry. He states that *when a tissue cell is resting, it will reject sodium and accept potassium. But when that same cell is active, it will accept sodium and reject potassium.*

So you would be wise to cut down on your sodium chloride intake and substitute potassium chloride or sea salt for your regular table salt instead. A *potassium gluconate* pill just before bedtime would certainly be advisable, too.

Insomnia Resulting from Specific Nutritional Deficiencies

Absence of this mineral catalyzer caused severe insomnia problems for Beatrice E. As I mentioned before, the lack of calcium can cause not only severe insomnia, but also other nervous symptoms that show up in the daytime as well. Beatrice was a patient with this problem.

When she came to see me, Beatrice was so nervous that no part of her body was ever completely still or at rest. She was constantly tapping her fingers, biting her nails, scratching her head, or crossing and uncrossing her legs. Beatrice was the best example of perpetual motion I have ever seen.

Beatrice told me she was extremely impatient with her family and snapped at them for no good reason. She was always restless, easily upset, and grouchy.

"I haven't had a decent night's sleep since heaven knows when," she said. "I wake up at the slightest noise, and then I can't go back to sleep. Every time my husband moves in bed it wakes me up; so we've started sleeping in different rooms so he won't disturb me. Every doctor I've been to says there's nothing wrong with me, that it's all in my head. But I know that's not true. For God's sake, please find out what's wrong so you can help me, doctor."

I immediately suspected Beatrice's insomnia and overly nervous problem to be a severe calcium deficiency, for one of the first major symptoms of a calcium shortage is extreme nervousness. Without calcium, the nerves cannot transmit messages properly. Muscles become tense and cannot relax.

A dietary analysis along with a laboratory test of a hair sample revealed that Beatrice was woefully deficient in her calcium intake. I immediately placed her on 3,000 milligrams of calcium in the form of dolomite along with 800 units of vitamin D to insure its proper absorption and utilization.

I also asked Beatrice to take 6 calcium lactate tablets with a small glass of warm milk just before going to bed to further help her insomnia. Milk contains tryptophan, an amino acid that induces sleep. Turkey contains huge amounts of tryptophan; this is one of the main reasons you feel so tired and sleepy after a big Thanksgiving dinner. The calcium in calcium lactate is quickly and readily absorbed, making it ideal as a "sleeping pill."

In only a few days, Beatrice was a completely changed woman. She became calm and serene. She slept so well without waking up that she and her husband are sleeping together again. Now with the ability to rest at night, Beatrice tells me she feels full of vigor and vitality. For her, calcium was the perfect catalytic health vitalizer.

HOW THIS POWERFUL CATALYTIC HEALTH VITALIZER CAN HELP YOU

I have found calcium to be outstanding in its ability to relieve nervous symptoms more quickly than perhaps anything else. For example, if your muscles become unexpectedly and suddenly weak and shaky, if your hands tremble when you're exerting yourself, if you feel weak and trembly in the legs, all you probably need is more calcium.

Or if you have children who have unpleasant dispositions, if they throw temper tantrums over nothing, if they constantly whimper and cry, give them some calcium. It'll do them more good than a spanking.

If you have already been taking calcium in a form other than dolomite—for example, bone meal—and still have problems sleeping, it could be that you have a shortage of magnesium. Let me explain that more fully. I once had a patient, Harriet T., who suffered from this problem. Harriet had read that calcium was good for insomnia (which is definitely true); so she had on her own been taking bone meal in mega-doses, but without results.

When I analyzed Harriet's diet, I found she had a severe shortage of magnesium, which can also cause nervous symptoms and insomnia just as can a deficiency of calcium. Harriet simply had no intake whatever of magnesium, for bone meal does not contain magnesium, but only phosphorus and calcium. Not only that, but in spite of all the calcium she had been taking in, she had a borderline calcium deficiency, too.

You see, when the body takes in too much phosphorus, as it was doing in Harriet's case, it must get rid of it. Since phosphorus and calcium are in combination, when phosphorus leaves the body, it takes calcium with it. Harriet was oversupplying her body with the phosphorus in bone meal. The excess phosphorus left her body, dragging calcium along with it, thus causing her borderline deficiency of this essential catalytic health energizer.

I simply changed Harriet's intake of calcium from bone meal to dolomite. When she took 2,000 milligrams of calcium in dolomite, she also got nearly 1,000 milligrams of magnesium. This simple change solved her insomnia problem immediately.

HOW THIS MAGIC MINERAL CATALYZER LULLED NORMAN I. TO SLEEP EASILY

Not all cases of insomnia are due to a calcium or magnesium deficiency. Some come from a shortage of a certain magic mineral catalytic health energizer which is often known as *nature's tranquilizer for the nervous system.* Let me use Norman's case history as an example of this.

Norman was extremely nervous and jumpy and had been taking prescription sleeping pills for quite a long time. However, his body had evidently adapted itself to them, for they were no longer as effective as they once were. After watching a television program that was highly critical of sleeping pills and tranquilizers, Norman decided to take a completely different approach to his insomnia problem.

My physical examination of Norman did not reveal any

specific difficulty that could be causing his insomnia. Nor could I discover any psychological problem in Norman's life that might be a contributing factor. However, the dietary analysis was a different story. Norman was badly deficient in the catalytic health vitalizer, zinc.

I put Norman on 60 milligrams of zinc each day for the first month, reducing it to 30 milligrams daily after that. The very first night Norman slept better than he ever had with all his sleeping pills. During the following weeks, his body completely eliminated the harmful effects of the tranquilizing drugs he had been taking, and his zinc became even more effective. Norman says he no longer has any problem whatever sleeping and that his energy levels are much higher than before.

WHAT THIS SAME MAGIC MINERAL
CAN DO FOR YOU

I was not at all surprised to hear Norman says his energy levels were higher, for zinc is not only nature's tranquilizer, but also one of nature's best vitalizers. It is necessary for the proper utilization of B-1 and B-12, both of which are energy supplying vitamins.

Zinc is also required for proper tissue respiration—the intake of oxygen and the expulsion of CO_2 and other toxic waste products. Zinc also improves brain activity to make a person more alert and mentally sharp. Finally, zinc is necessary for proper carbohydrate metabolism to produce abundant body energy.

If you have an energy lack, or if you have insomnia, take 30 milligrams of zinc each day. It could easily solve both your problems.

Other Factors That Relieve
Insomnia Quickly and Safely

THE SLEEP VITAMINS:
VITAMIN C AND INOSITOL

I never cease to be amazed at the versatility of Nature. She wastes nothing. She can use a vitamin to increase energy levels and at the same time use that same vitamin as a tranquilizer to help a person sleep and rest better.

Vitamin C is one example of this. Mega-doses of vitamin C have an anti-anxiety or sedative effect on the human nervous system. The effect of a large dose lasts for 6 to 8 hours. Therefore, a wise procedure would be to take at least 2,000 milligrams of vitamin C just before going to bed.

Inositol, one of the B vitamins, is another catalytic health vitalizer that can be used as a sedative at bedtime. Two-thousand milligrams could be the answer for your problem of insomnia. I have used Inositol successfully with many of my patients.

CLIFF F. FINDS THIS NATURAL TRANQUILIZER TO BE MOST EFFECTIVE FOR HIM

Admittedly, this business of finding the exact cure for insomnia can be most difficult at times. This is especially true when no dietary deficiency exists or when no emotional problem can be found. Cliff F. was one such patient. Finally, as a last resort, I asked Cliff to try some *chamomile tea*. This was his answer. It worked like a charm.

Cliff would make a cup of chamomile tea, add a teaspoon of honey, and drink it just before going to bed. It calmed his nerves and let him drop off into a sound sleep soon after lying down.

How good is chamomile tea as a sleep-inducer? Well, a group of medical doctors found that it worked wonders for cardiac patients who had undergone ventricular catheterization. Drinking the chamomile tea had no effect on the person's heart. But 10 out of 12 patients who drank the tea dropped off soon afterward into a deep hypnotic-like sleep.

If chamomile tea could make a person fall asleep immediately after undergoing such a painful anxiety-producing procedure as catheterization of the heart, it surely ought to perform miracles for the person with insomnia.

If you happen to be that person, chamomile tea could be the answer for you, just as it was for Cliff. It soothes the nerves, relaxes the body, acts as a sedative, and unlike sleeping pills, is completely harmless. Try it; you have nothing to lose but your insomnia.

Insomnia Caused by Emotional or Mental Problems

Fear, anxiety, and worry can cause insomnia just as can specific nutritional deficiencies. In such a situation, I would suggest you take some of the catalytic health vitalizers mentioned in the final subsection of this chapter. Even though these may not specifically cure your insomnia if it is caused by mental or emotional problems, they will help take the edge off your jagged nerves.

I know that if you have financial worries, marital problems, or other conditions in your life that cause anxiety and fear, you cannot just snap your fingers and make them go away. However, I do have several techniques that have helped a lot of people out of the deep valleys of depression and despair. These guidelines will not necessarily solve your basic emotional problem, but they could help you gain enough serenity and peace of mind to see your problem clearly enough to solve it. Do that, and then you can sleep.

1. *Live Only in the Ever-Present Now.* If you live in yesterday or tomorrow, you cannot help but have emotional problems or suffer psychological trauma. The following thoughts about yesterday, tomorrow, and today should prove extremely useful to you:

Yesterday. There are 2 days in every week about which you should not worry, 2 days which should be kept free from fear and apprehension. One of these days is yesterday, with its mistakes and cares, its faults and blunders, its aches and pains. Yesterday has passed forever beyond your control. All the money in the world cannot bring back yesterday. You cannot undo a single act you performed. You cannot erase a single word you said. Yesterday is gone forever beyond recall.

160

Tomorrow. The other day you should not worry about is tomorrow, with its possible adversities, its burdens, its large promises and perhaps its poor performance. Tomorrow is also beyond your immediate control. Tomorrow's sun will rise, either in splendor or behind a mask of clouds; but it will rise. Until it does, you have no stake in tomorrow, for it is yet unborn.

Today. This leaves only one day for you to worry about—today. Anyone can fight the battles of just one day. It is only when you and I add the burden of those 2 awful eternities, yesterday and tomorrow, that we break down. It is not the experience of today that drives one mad. It is the remorse or the bitterness for something which happened yesterday or the dread of what tomorrow might bring. Therefore, do your best to live just one day at a time.

I am indebted for the above thoughts about yesterday, tomorrow, and today to one of my patients who is a member of Alcoholics Anonymous. He gave me a card they use in A. A. with these ideas on it. It had no author indicated; so I cannot give credit to anyone, but I'm sure the individual must have been an extremely wise person.

2. *Do Your Worrying at the Right Time.* If you must worry, then worry at the right time of day. You can't solve a single problem by worrying about it after you go to bed. If you find yourself worrying about something after you've retired for the night, toll yourself that *night time is for sleeping.* If you really do have something worth while to worry about, then *think about your problem during the day when you can do something constructive about it.* Many of my patients with insomnia tell me they have solved their problem completely with this simple approach.

In the Final Analysis

If you cannot isolate the specific cause of your insomnia from the preceding information, then I would suggest you take the following catalytic health vitalizers about a half hour or so before going to bed. I know they will be of help to you.

1. 1,000 milligrams of *calcium* in the form of dolomite,
2. *Magnesium*, which is automatically included in dolomite,
3. 30 milligrams of *zinc*,
4. 200 to 400 units of *vitamin E*,
5. 2,000 to 3,000 milligrams of *vitamin C*,
6. 2,000 milligrams of *Inositol*,
7. One *potassium gluconate* pill, and
8. One cup of *chamomile tea* or one *small* glass of *warm milk* with a teaspoon of *honey*.

If after all this you still can't sleep, then as a last resort I would suggest you use the method my wife's sister uses. She simply lies down when she is sleepy—day or night—and sleeps, period; sometimes for 15 minutes, sometimes for an hour. If she wakes up at night, she does not lie in bed worrying about it. She gets up, makes a pot of tea, scrambles some eggs, reads a book, plays the piano or organ. When she is tired and sleepy again, she goes back to bed.

I know you can't always do this, especially if you work at a 9 to 5 job, have children to send off to school, a husband to cook meals for, and so on. But if you're down to just 2 of you in the house, retired, and with no other responsibilities to fulfill, why not try it?

Don't worry about what people might say or think. Do what you want to do, not what your neighbors or your friends or your children *think* you ought to do. You are not responsible for what other people *think*. That's their problem; don't make it yours.

11

How Certain Catalytic Health Vitalizers Can Refresh and Heal Tired and Jagged Nerves

Although you have already met most of the catalytic health vitalizers I will discuss in this chapter, I now want to tell you how they can be used to relieve neuritis, neuralgia, depression, nervous ailments such as petit mal and epilepsy, and finally, just "plain old nerves."

How This Potent Health Vitalizer Relieved Beulah K's Neuralgia

Beulah had been bothered with facial neuralgia for several months. She suffered with an intense stabbing and burning pain on the left side of her face that ran from her temple down across the cheek to her chin.

The painful neuralgia attacks would be precipitated by extremely minor events—for example, eating hot or cold foods, drinking a cup of hot coffee or a glass of cold water, a sudden cold draft on the face, or an unexpected bumping or jarring of the body. Even washing her face could cause an attack.

Not only was the attack of neuralgia painful to Beulah, but it was also accompanied by such irritating symptoms as twitching of the left side of her face, watering of the eye and nostril on that side, and a drooping of the left corner of her mouth.

Medication to prevent the attacks had proved to be ineffective; so Beulah's doctor had recommended surgical intervention. However, Beulah did not want to resort to such a drastic procedure unless it was absolutely necessary.

X-rays of Beulah's neck showed some cervical misalignment that was quickly and easily corrected. This reduced both the frequency and severity of her attacks, but it did not eliminate them altogether. An analysis of Beulah's dietary intake revealed that she was extremely deficient in the vitamin B complex, which is not at all uncommon in a great many nervous conditions.

I placed Beulah on a high B complex supplement. I also gave her an additional amount of vitamin B-12 (250 micrograms) per day, which is extremely effective in such cases. Her relief was almost like a miracle. In less than 10 days she was completely free of her painful attacks of neuralgia. She has continued to take her vitamin B complex each day along with the extra B-12 for the past 6 months and has had no recurrence of her problem.

Beulah also tells me her energy reserves are much higher than before. She used to tire easily and was ready to go back to bed a couple of hours after she got up in the morning. Now she says she can go all day without any trouble at all.

Larry V's Psychosis Completely Cured

Although I am not a psychiatrist or a psychologist, I have always been deeply interested in all kinds of nervous diseases. In recent years, megavitamin therapy for such conditions as schizophrenia, paranoia, and mental depression has achieved spectacular results. When Larry's mother, Ida V., brought him to me for a paranoia-like psychosis, I decided to use the marvelous catalytic health vitalizer B-12 for his treatment.

Larry was 12 years old. He had been sent home from a boy scout summer encampment because of his behavior. At home, he was irritable, moody, and suspicious of everyone. He claimed that people, even his parents and brothers and sisters, were all talking about him and saying bad things about him behind his back. Upon passing a complete stranger in the street, he would say he knew that individual hated him for he could tell by the expression on his face.

For his psychotic condition, Larry's previous doctor had prescribed one of the phenothiazine drugs, specifically trifluoperazine, which is often used for psychotic behavior. However, Larry's mother was not at all satisfied with this procedure and brought him to me.

I gave Larry 150 micrograms of B-12 (75 micrograms twice a day in tablet form) along with a high potency B-complex for proper balance. The results were little short of miraculous. In less than 4 weeks, Larry's delusions and hallucinations had ceased altogether. He no longer felt persecuted or that everyone was plotting against him. His mother says it's like having a different boy in the house now. She used to dread seeing him come home from school, but not any more.

Larry's improvement has been maintained more than a year and a half now with vitamin B-12 and the high-potency B complex. We have double-checked and experimented several times to see if the vitamin therapy was actually the reason for Larry's improvement. We did this by discontinuing his dosage for a few days. His psychotic symptoms would return immediately; so there is no doubt in our minds any longer that the vitamin B complex with extra B-12 is the best treatment for Larry's condition.

How This Amazing Catalytic Health Vitalizer
Improved Carol L's School Work

Carol's mother, Donna, brought her to me because of her mental attitude and her low grades in school. Carol's teacher had told Donna that Carol was much slower in grasping new ideas than the other students. She was also sullen and uncooperative. In fact, the teacher was concerned that Carol might be mentally retarded.

Carol had difficulty with time perception and logical thought processes. When she closed her eyes, she said she often continued to see strange things and hear odd sounds. Most of the time, she seemed completely disoriented and out of touch with her actual surroundings. There was no doubt in my mind that Carol had a nervous problem, for other than being slightly underweight she seemed quite well physically.

I recommended vitamin B-12 for Carol (300 micrograms divided into 3 daily doses of 100 micrograms each), along with a high potency vitamin B supplement for proper balance. I also asked Carol's mother to keep her on a high-protein, low-sugar diet.

The fantastic results were not only noticed by Carol's mother, but also by her school teacher, who said there was a great improvement in Carol's behavior and her attitude toward her school work. The teacher also said Carol had a far greater interest in all school activities and a much longer attention span than before.

Donna was most gratified to see her daughter's grades go from D's and F's up to A's and B's. Carol also gained weight and felt much better in general than before.

How Carl J's Troublesome Neuritis
Was Completely Resolved

Carl had been bothered for some time with a painful neuritis in both legs. His calves were extremely tender, the muscles were weak, and he was troubled with cramps and tingling sensations from the feet clear up to his knees. At times his feet would swell and puff up so badly that he could not even get his shoes on.

Since Carl's symptoms were in both legs, I immediately suspected a diet deficiency. Had only one leg been affected, there would have been a greater possibility of a localized neuritis which could have been caused by a misalignment of the vertebrae in the lower part of the spine. But this was not the case.

A laboratory report of a hair sample for mineral content revealed no major deficiency; so I made a vitamin analysis of Carl's diet and found that he was extremely deficient in the vitamin B complex. Admittedly, it is difficult for any doctor to differentially diagnose and determine which factor of the B complex is missing or deficient in nervous conditions, but from past experience I was sure that Carl needed more thiamine (B-1). I have almost always found it to be missing in severe cases of neuritis.

I placed Carl on 1,000 milligrams of thiamine daily. Of course I also had him take the complete B complex for proper balance. Carl responded quickly to his treatment and was relieved of all his symptoms in less than a month. As long as he continues his vitamin B supplementation, he has no problem whatever with the neuritis in his legs.

Carl tells me he also feels much more mentally alert than before and that he seems to have an unlimited supply of energy. As he so aptly put it, "Boy, Doc, I feel so good I can hardly believe it!"

How This Phenomenal Catalytic Health Vitalizer Overcame Ruth U's Severe Nervous Depression

Ruth had been hospitalized for a complete nervous breakdown before she came to see me. She had fallen into a deep depression, had lost all interest in life, and was extremely nervous, unable to relax, or to sleep at night. This depression persisted almost all the time, although Ruth's husband, Gordon, said that occasionally her moods would swing to periods of elation, almost as if she were "high" on drugs.

During these rare periods she would bustle about the house, cleaning and scrubbing vigorously as if she were doing an old-fashioned spring or fall house cleaning. At those times she seemed to have unlimited pep and energy.

Unfortunately, right in the middle of all this frenzied activity she would suddenly fall into a period of depression again and go immediately to her bedroom. As a result, the house would often be left in a complete mess with closets emptied and clothes scattered all over the room or buckets of dirty water left standing in the kitchen or the utility room.

However, most of the time Ruth stayed in the bedroom just sitting in a chair staring out the window or lying down on the bed. She always had "the blues" and complained that everything seemed to be just "too much for her to handle" and that nothing in life was at all worth while. She had a constant feeling of impending doom along with an extreme fear of dying. She didn't want to be left alone, yet she could not tolerate her daughters or her husband when they were in the bedroom with her.

Ruth was not able to do the ordinary daily chores around the house or even cook a meal for her family; so all the household duties had fallen on Gordon and the 2 daughters.

Her doctor had recommended that Ruth be placed in a mental institution for observation and possible electric shock therapy, but Gordon said he would not consider this procedure under any circumstances whatever.

Shortly before Ruth came to my office, Gordon had been reading about megavitamin therapy for emotional and nervous problems, and for the first time since she'd been sick, it occurred to them that her problem might possibly be due to a dietary deficiency of some sort.

Since a lack of *biotin* (a B complex factor) is primarily responsible for causing a depression and lassitude similar to Ruth's condition, I decided on that approach. I gave her 300 micrograms of biotin daily along with a high potency balanced B complex.

I also asked Ruth to eat a high-protein low-sugar diet, for I have found that refined white sugar by itself can be responsible for a great many nervous ailments. Not only that, but refined white sugar actually causes a deficiency of the vitamin B complex in the body. This results in abnormally slow tissue metabolism leaving incompletely oxidized toxic products in the blood stream. This is not only bad for the nervous system, but also for the heart.

In only 2 weeks, Ruth was much better. She became calmer and far less nervous than before. She began to take an active interest in her surroundings again. In only 3 months, she and her family were back to normal. Ruth was doing her own housework, cooking the meals, and taking care of the grocery shopping as well. As Gordon said, she was a completely changed woman, full of pep and energy, with no personality hang-ups. What a wonderful catalytic health vitalizer the vitamin B complex is for nervous conditions such as Ruth had.

I would like to point out here that one does not necessarily have to be deficient in a particular vitamin to have it be of benefit. In mental and nervous conditions especially, it seems that many times the patient has been born deficient in a certain critical body enzyme.

The reason the B complex of vitamins is so useful in problems of mental disorientation is because all the B vitamins, with the exception of choline, function as coenzymes in the body. The coenzyme is one of the main parts of a body enzyme; so without enough of the B complex, sufficient enzymes cannot be formed to carry out many of the body's vital functions, particularly in the nervous system.

How Eddie B's Petit Mal
Was Cleared Up As if by Magic

Eddie was troubled with *petit mal* (a form of epilepsy) for almost 2 years. He would suffer from 3 to 4 seizures a day. During these attacks, his face would go blank, his eyes would roll, and his head would droop down. If the seizure was extremely severe, he would have convulsions with an occasional loss of bowel and bladder control.

Although the petit mal kind of epilepsy is not considered as dangerous as *grand mal*, primarily because in the grand mal type the person has violent convulsions, usually falling on the ground and rolling around, still the individual can suffer injury during this period of transitory unconsciousness, or he can cause severe damage to others.

After the attack was over, Eddie would have no recollection whatever of it, and he would go on with whatever he was doing as if nothing unusual had happened.

Eddie was only 4 at this time, and his mother dreaded the thought of the day he would have to go to school. She was extremely anxious to get his condition corrected before then.

His seizures were not relieved by anti-convulsant therapy, and as so many people do when drugs do not work to cure an illness, Eddie's mother brought him to me as a last resort. I was sure that Eddie had to be deficient in the vitamin B complex, and since it was difficult for him to swallow a tablet or capsule, I had his mother give him 3 tablespoons of brewer's yeast in orange juice daily on a trial basis, for I knew it could not possibly hurt him.

Eddie's condition improved immediately; so I knew we were on the right track. I wanted to get him on vitamin B-6 (pyridoxine) supplementation as soon as possible, for B-6 is close to being a specific for epilepsy. With a lot of patience and coaxing and the promise of a reward afterward, we were finally able to get Eddie to swallow the B-6 tablets. I asked his mother to make sure he got 250 milligrams 3 times a day for a total of 750 milligrams.

Two weeks after the B-6 treatment was started, Eddie's seizures, which had already become milder and less frequent with the brewer's yeast, ceased altogether. I am happy to report that Eddie is now 7 years old, doing well in school, and has had no problem at all during all this time.

I'm sure he'll need to take the vitamin B supplementation all his life, for evidently Eddie is one of those born with a natural enzyme deficiency. But how much better vitamin B is than the anti-convulsant drugs that 2 neurologists insisted he would have to take as long as he lived. After all, vitamin B is a natural food, not a drug, and there are no dangerous side effects from its use.

Not only that, but where anti-convulsant drugs usually depress a person's nervous system to make him less responsive to external stimuli and thus more drowsy and sleepy, vitamin B supplies a person with a tremendous reserve supply of energy. Eddie's mother has noticed that he is much more alert and physically active than most children his age.

How This Remarkable Catalytic Health Vitalizer Can Help You, Too

If you are troubled with nervous problems of any sort, it could well be that the vitamin B complex will help you just as it has helped so many of my patients. Although it is always best to take the entire B complex, if you do have certain specific nervous conditions you should also take the various individual B factors I have indicated below:

For instance, if you have neuritis, you would be wise to take additional thiamine (B-1). At least 1,000 milligrams a day is considered to be a therapeutic dose for neuritis. Thiamine is also useful in treating non-specific mental illnesses, sciatica, and multiple sclerosis.

Nervous disorders such as Parkinson's disease and multiple sclerosis are also treated with vitamin B-2 (riboflavin). Doctors specializing in megavitamin therapy recommend at least 1,000 milligrams every day.

Niacin (vitamin B-3) has been used successfully in any number of nervous conditions, for example, paranoia, schizophrenia, depression, anxiety neurosis, hyperactivity in children, mental retardation, and alcoholism. It has also been found useful in some cases of Parkinson's disease, epilepsy, and multiple sclerosis. The usual recommended daily dosage for such conditions is from 1,500 to 3,000 milligrams.

Vitamin B-6 (pyridoxine) can be valuable in epilepsy, mental illness, neuritis, Parkinson's disease, multiple sclerosis, and Bell's palsy. The recommended therapeutic dose is 750 milligrams daily.

A deficiency of B-12 causes a variety of nervous and muscular symptoms. I have achieved some stunning results with its use. If you are troubled with any of the following problems that have not responded to other measures, take 250 *micrograms* (not milligrams) of B-12 each day. You could easily see your problem dissolve into thin air. A B-12 deficiency can cause any or all of the following:

1. Subtle, unexplained changes in your nervous system and mental attitudes,

2. Soreness and weakness in your arms and legs,

3. Difficulties in walking,

4. Involuntary jerking of the limbs,

5. Diminished reflexes and sensory perception,

6. Changes in temperature in different parts of the body.

Even if you eat bread and cereals enriched with the B vitamins, you will still need additional supplementation for the treatment of nervous conditions. Enrichment of bread and cereals is in extremely minute quantities. Megavitamin therapy is needed in nervous ailments to get the desired results.

If you are taking medicines or drugs of any sort, especially an antibiotic such as penicillin, you would be wise to supplement your diet with plenty of the energy producing vitamin B complex. Drugs and medicines, particularly the antibiotics, leave a person drained of energy, pale, without any appetite, constipated or diarrhetic, nervous and jumpy, cross and cranky, and in short, terribly difficult to live with. A high potency B complex can help prevent these problems even before they happen.

Although many of the factors of the B complex are important in treating mental and nervous problems, other catalytic health vitalizers are valuable, too. I'd like to discuss some of them now.

How Betty Z's Nervous Problems Were Easily Resolved with This Incredible Treatment

Betty had been taking nerve tranquilizers and sedatives for the past 5 years when she came to see me. Several doctors had told her that her nervous problems were only emotional and that she needed psychiatric care.

Unless she had a tranquilizing drug 3 or 4 times a day, Betty simply could not function at all. She had an almost overwhelming sense of anxiety and nervousness. Simple social situations terrified her. She was also unable to make a decision of any sort.

One of her friends, a patient of mine, suggested that perhaps her problem was physiological rather than psychological and recommended that she come to my office.

Betty's physical examination revealed that she was 10 to 12 pounds underweight. Her face showed the effects of her nervous condition, for it was pale and haggard, and perpetual frown lines creased her forehead. Her nails had been bitten down to the quick, and she told me that sometimes she chewed on them until her fingers actually bled.

The clue to what was basically wrong with Betty was found in a mineral analysis of her hair. She was highly deficient in zinc. I was not at all surprised to find this, for if you will remember, I mentioned in the last chapter that zinc is known as *nature's tranquilizer for the nervous system.*

I started Betty on 60 milligrams of zinc gluconate and continued this treatment for 30 days. At the end of only 2 weeks, Betty had made amazing progress. In fact, her recovery was almost like a miracle. She was no longer nervous and jumpy. She was calm, collected, and completely at ease in the presence of others. She was now able to make decisions without hesitation.

I sent in a second hair sample to the laboratory at the end of the first month of treatment. The report showed that her body's zinc levels had risen approximately 60 percent. We then reduced her intake to 30 milligrams each day. A third hair sample at the end of the third month revealed that her zinc content was normal.

Betty hasn't taken a tranquilizer or sedative for more than a year now. The lines are gone from her face, and her weight is now normal for her height and age. She still takes 30 milligrams of zinc each day, for, as she says, she doesn't want to run the risk of her nervous condition coming back again. Betty also tells me she feels much more alive, alert, and energetic than she has in many, many years. Zinc gluconate was the perfect catalytic health vitalizer for her.

How This Catalytic Health Vitalizer Can Be of Benefit to You

To best show you how this catalytic health vitalizer, zinc, can help you, let me tell you what it has done for others. For example, recent research has shown that school children with poor appetites, slow growth rates, and a subnormal sense of taste and smell suffer from a zinc deficiency. This has also been found to be the case with lethargic pupils who were apathetic about their school work. In an experiment conducted at the University of Michigan, students' hair samples were tested for trace minerals. Those with the highest academic grades had more zinc in their systems than those with lower grades. Dr. Robert I. Henken of the National Heart and Lung Institute says that zinc supplements have effectively restored the sense of taste and smell in over 100 patients. So if you suffer with any of these problems, take 30 milligrams of zinc gluconate daily. I know you'll be most happy that you did.

How Lucy N's "Anxiety Neurosis" Was Healed in Only Three Short Weeks

Lucy suffered from what psychiatrists call an *anxiety neurosis*. She slept badly, had no appetite, and had a constant feeling of impending doom as if something terrible was about to happen. As Lucy told me, "I get all uptight for no good reason at all. I always feel like I have a heavy lump of dough in my stomach. I get all sweaty, my hands feel clammy, and it's hard for me to breathe—just as if I'm about to have a heart attack. I'm afraid of the light; I'm afraid of the dark; I'm afraid of people, but I'm scared to be alone. In fact, I'm afraid of everything!"

I suspected a calcium, magnesium, or zinc deficiency in Lucy's case. A hair sample revealed by laboratory analysis that she was extremely deficient in calcium. I put Lucy on 5,000 milligrams of calcium each day in the form of dolomite, and in only 3 weeks she felt completely normal again. All her symptoms simply disappeared.

After 3 months of feeling good, Lucy suddenly became skeptical of her treatment. She found it hard to believe that a mere change in her diet could be responsible for so quick and dramatic an improvement. So without my knowledge, she stopped taking her dolomite. In only 3 days all her old symptoms returned. Lucy needed no more convincing. She started taking her dolomite again and has not experimented since.

Other Ways in Which a Shortage of This Catalytic Vitalizer Affects People

Calcium deficiencies generally sneak up slowly on a person. Usually, the body protects itself from low blood levels of calcium by drawing upon bone and muscle reserves. But the nervous system cannot go on *stealing* calcium indefinitely from body tissues. Eventually the calcium balance must be restored if health is to be maintained.

Just a tiny decrease in the blood can produce uncontrollable temper outbursts. Young children are extremely vulnerable. Babies will hold their breath and turn blue; toddlers often have outrageous tempers. If a youngster tends to have tantrums for no reason, consider a calcium deficiency. That will usually be the answer for such unwarranted behavior in youngsters.

What This Catalytic Health Vitalizer Can Do for "Plain Old Nerves"

When too little calcium is circulating in the blood stream to spark the nervous system, palpitation and racing of the heart, sweating, and "plain old nerves" are the natural end result. I have used calcium successfully on a great many cases of plain old nerves when other doctors have said it was "all in the person's head."

Sometimes a woman will break down and cry for no apparent

reason at all that a man can see. And she won't be able to give a good explanation why except that her nerves are jagged and on edge. A lot of doctors will says she's neurotic and that there's nothing wrong with her, but they're mistaken. I know that 99 times out of 100 she's not neurotic at all. She's deficient in calcium, and that's what her body is crying for.

So if your problem is "plain old nerves," and your doctor insists that you're not really sick at all, do this: Take some calcium in the form of dolomite every day, at least 2,000 milligrams. It can't hurt you in any way at all. It would also be wise to take at least 400 units of vitamin D to insure absorption and utilization of the calcium. Add 30 milligrams of zinc on a daily basis. Then take a high potency B complex along with some desiccated liver and brewer's yeast. So help me, if you don't feel better, well . . . but then, I know that you will, for I've seen it happen time after time after time.

Or if you have a magnesium deficiency, as so many people do, dolomite will solve those problems, too. Dr. Willard A. Krehl of the University of Iowa, analyzing a group of patients with mild magnesium deficiencies, found that 22 percent had convulsions; 44 percent suffered hallucinations; 78 percent evidenced mental confusion; 83 percent were disoriented and couldn't remember where they were. They didn't recall the year, the day, the month, or the time of day. One-hundred percent startled easily and were alarmed by unexpected movement and noise.

Since both magnesium and calcium are needed for proper nerve conduction, muscular contraction, and the transmission of impulses all along the nervous system, it doesn't matter which one is deficient (although chances are both of them will be); dolomite will solve the problem for you, since it contains both calcium and magnesium in the proper proportions.

12

How You Can Whip the Exhaustion Caused by Digestive Troubles with These Superb Catalytic Health Vitalizers

Although many problems are associated with the digestive tract, in this chapter I will discuss those that I encounter most often in my practice. I see no point in talking about some exotic intestinal disease that exists primarily in a textbook. Not only that, but the ailments I will cover cause not only pain and discomfort, but also excessive exhaustion and fatigue. Diarrhea, for example, can give you that washed-out, dragged-down feeling more quickly than almost anything I know of.

So you're going to read about common conditions for which

I'm sure you've used over-the-counter, non-prescription remedies many, many times in the past (for instance: diarrhea, constipation, hemorrhoids, canker sores, and indigestion).

You're going to discover some new and much more efficient remedies for those conditions. The superb catalytic health vitalizers I'll describe can eliminate these problems for you quickly and easily, allowing you to regain your strength and energy, your vigor and vitality.

How Fred P. Got Rid of His Chronic Constipation Quickly and Easily Without Harsh Laxatives

Fred did not come to me for his constipation problem, but for a different ailment entirely. However, during the process of taking his past health history, this condition came to light. Naturally, he wanted to get rid of it if he could.

Fred had been bothered with poor elimination for more than 20 years. He had gone to many doctors during that time, but none of them had ever found a permanent cure for his constipation. Fred usually had only one bowel movement every 4 or 5 days. Sometimes he went even longer. His stools were exceptionally hard, and his bowel movements were extremely painful. Fred had used every artificial laxative he'd ever heard of or read about. None of them had ever given him any permanent or lasting relief.

I found Fred to be very deficient in his vitamin B intake. I asked him to take one tablespoon of brewer's yeast in a glass of fruit juice before each meal, and amazingly, his constipation vanished in only 3 days. Fred has been taking brewer's yeast 3 times a day now for the past 6 months and has had no more trouble at all.

The elimination of his constipation has done wonders for Fred in many other ways. Where before he felt dumpy and loggy all the time and had no ambition to do anything, he now feels vigorous and full of energy, ready to tackle any job.

Fred's wife, Gladys, tells me the brewer's yeast has changed his disposition completely. She says he used to be grouchy and irritable, but now he is pleasant and easy to get along with.

Brewer's yeast was the perfect catalytic health vitalizer for Fred; 20 years of problems literally went down the drain almost overnight.

How You Can Benefit
from Fred's Case History

Most people think the greatest danger of constipation is the absorption of toxic products back into the body. Actually, the greatest danger is the use of harsh laxatives and cathartics that irritate delicate intestinal mucous membranes and interfere with digestion and absorption.

Mineral oil, probably the most damaging of all laxatives, decreases the absorption and assimilation of calcium and phosphorus. It absorbs the fat-soluble vitamins A, D, E, and K, and carries them out of the body in the stools. If you're now spending money on vitamins A, D, and E, and then taking mineral oil for constipation at the same time, you'd be better off spending that vitamin money on a movie. At least you'd get some value and enjoyment out of it, for you're not getting any return at all from your investment in vitamins, and you won't until you stop taking mineral oil.

Brewer's yeast could well be the answer for you as it has been for Fred and so many of my patients. However, I would highly recommend you use what my patients call the *Three-B Program*. Before I discuss that, let me tell you what kind of a problem constipation really is. Then you'll better understand why I use the 3-B Program and why it is so successful.

Constipation is actually caused by 2 major factors. First is the lack of a chemical-nervo-stimulus resulting from an insufficient vitamin B intake. That's why brewer's yeast works so well in most cases. The second factor is the retention of *low-residue* waste products in the large intestine for too long a period of time. The large intestine has 2 major functions. One is to move the waste out of the body. The other is to conserve water. The longer the waste matter remains in the body, the more water will be withdrawn, and the harder the stools will become.

179

Since man-made packaged and processed foods have no bulk and very little residue, the large intestine has nothing to move along when those foods are eaten. There must be bulk in the diet, or there will be constipation. It's as simple as that.

Unless a patient has some intestinal anatomical abnormality, I can say without hesitation that a lack of the vitamin B complex for chemical-nervo-stimulus and modern, civilized, packaged, man-made foods without the necessary bulk for physical stimulus are the exact causes of constipation in every single case I have ever treated.

How a Low-Residue Diet
Causes Constipation

How does a low-residue diet of man-made foods produce constipation? How do bulk, roughage, and indigestible fiber work to prevent constipation? Here's how: Waste matter is normally moved along the intestines by waves of muscular contraction. When the bowels are relatively full of waste matter, the muscles surrounding the membrane lining of the intestines need to contract only slightly to move it along. But when waste matter is scanty and compacted, as it is in those eating a highly refined diet of man-made foods, the muscles have to contract with much greater force to create the pressure needed to keep things moving.

It is much like squeezing a tube of toothpaste. When the tube is full or nearly full, only a slight pressure is needed to expel the toothpaste. But when the tube is nearly empty, you have to squeeze and squeeze harder and harder to get the contents out. That's exactly what you do when you strain at the stool. You squeeze harder and harder to get the waste material out.

How the Three-B Program Will
Get Rid of Your Constipation

The Three-B Program consists of the vitamin B complex, Brewer's yeast, and unprocessed Bran. I almost always have a patient with constipation take the B vitamin complex, brewer's yeast, and 2 to 3 tablespoons of unprocessed bran each day.

The vitamin B complex and brewer's yeast, which also contains the full complex of B vitamins in their natural state, are important in restoring the strength and tone to the muscles of the digestive tract. They provide the chemical-nervo stimulus that is needed. Keep in mind that your nerves move the muscles of the bowels, and they will do this for you only if your vitamin B intake is sufficient. I also ask my patients with constipation to take desiccated liver since this is also a potent, natural source of the vitamin B complex. If you are constipated, you cannot get too much vitamin B.

Unprocessed bran is important for a person suffering with constipation, for it helps absorb moisture and maintain bulk in the digestive system. The retention of moisture is important, for it keeps the person from suffering unnecessary discomfort from hard dry stools.

Two to 3 tablespoons of unprocessed bran each day are usually enough. Most of my patients mix the bran with other cereal or use it in hamburger, meat loaf, and so on. All-Bran, which is available in the supermarket, will also provide bulk in your stool, but I by far prefer the unprocessed bran that you get in the health food store, for it has no sugar or other artificial additives.

I also ask my patients to avoid man-made products such as doughnuts, rolls, white bread, and the like. These contain bleached white flour and are particularly troublesome for white flour has no bulk or fiber at all. I consider white bread as perhaps the greatest offender here. It stops the bowels almost as effectively as if the person had swallowed a cup of glue.

Many manufacturers today are finally recognizing the public's desire for high fiber natural breads. That's why you see so many more loaves of whole wheat bread, 7 grain breads, and high fiber bran breads on the shelves in the grocery store.

So you would be wise to choose one of these high fiber breads instead of white bread. You can also get whole grain cereals instead of the ones you see advertised every Saturday morning on TV. Fresh vegetables and fruits—eaten raw if possible—are to be preferred over canned ones.

To sum if up, then, you can easily and quickly get over your constipation, no matter how long you've had it, if you will follow these few simple guidelines faithfully:

1. Take a high potency vitamin B complex every day.
2. Take 3 tablespoons of brewer's yeast each day, one before each meal in fruit juice.
3. Use 2 to 3 tablespoons of unprocessed bran every day. Mix it in your other cereals, hamburger, meat loaf, and so on.
4. Eat fresh fruit and vegetables, raw if possible.
5. Eat foods that are born, not made.
6. Use stone-ground 100 percent whole wheat bread or a high fiber bread. Eat whole grain cereals.
7. Avoid those man-made foods that contain bleached white flour. It has no fiber or bulk whatever.

Statistical Benefits of the Three-B Program

How effective is this Three-B Program? Well, to show you that, I reviewed 100 case histories of constipation that I have treated in my office. Before going on my Three-B Program, 86 patients strained at the stool all the time. Fourteen strained most of the time. None of them could have a bowel movement without some difficulty and effort. None of them had a bowel movement every day. Most of them went only every third or fourth day.

After going on the Three-B Program, all of them had at least 1 bowel movement every day. Most of them had 2. All of them had normal stools. And without exception, all these patients felt better. They had more strength and energy, more vigor and vitality. One of these patients summed it up this way: "Doc, if I didn't know how old I was, I'd swear I was back in my teens again. What a wonderful sensation it is to be healthy and regular and feel energetic and full of life for a change!"

How Eileen T's Hemorrhoids Were Relieved with This Fantastic Catalytic Health Vitalizer

Before I tell you about Eileen's case, I want to say that every case of chronic constipation will eventually bring on hemorrhoids because of straining and bearing down at the stool. The more you strain and bear down, the sooner the hemorrhoids will appear. Pregnancy, as in Eileen's case, simply speeds up their arrival.

Eileen had for quite some time been bothered with constipation. But she did not come to me for that. She came to see if I could help her hemorrhoids. She had used various medications, ointments, and rectal suppositories including the popular brands you see advertised on TV and in magazines and newspapers all the time. No permanent relief had been obtained. The blood vessel walls surrounding the anal opening were so thin that cleansing after a bowel movement would cause them to bleed. Besides the pain and bleeding, her hemorrhoids itched badly. This caused Eileen a great deal of discomfort.

However, as I told Eileen, before we could clear up the hemorrhoids we had to resolve her constipation problem. I placed her on my 3-B program for that. In less than one week, her bowel movements were normal. We then concentrated our attention on her hemorrhoids.

I had previously learned that vitamin E inserts had been used successfully in Canada for both hemorrhoids and atrophic vaginitis, so I decided to use that approach. After all, hemorrhoids are varicose veins, and I knew that vitamin E helped varicose veins and so would help Eileen's hemorrhoids.

Since I had no vitamin E inserts (they are not available in the United States, at least in my area), I had Eileen use a vitamin E capsule as a suppository after each bowel movement. She used the one containing 400 international units. I also asked her to take 1,200 units of vitamin E each day orally to strengthen her entire blood vascular system.

Eileen responded quite rapidly to her treatment. In only 2

weeks the condition was nearly cleared up. However, because of the thinness of the blood vessel walls, she still uses extreme care in cleansing herself after a bowel movement.

Now that her constipation is gone and no further damage is caused to those blood vessels by hard bowel movements, the vitamin E will in time build up their muscular tone and elasticity. I cannot say for sure that they will return completely to normal, but I can say that Eileen no longer suffers any ill effects of any sort from her hemorrhoids.

What You Can Do for Hemorrhoids Yourself

Of course, the first thing to do is to get rid of the constipation problem if it exists. Next, I would suggest that you be very careful not to use coarse toilet paper. I ask my patients who have extremely severe hemorrhoids to first cleanse themselves gently with soft toilet paper and then to finish the cleansing process with a sponge and warm water. This will prevent tearing and opening up of the thin walls of the injured blood vessels.

Vitamin E suppositories—known commercially as "Vitamin E Inserts"—have been on the market in Canada for some years now and have been used successfully for both hemorrhoids and atrophic vaginitis. However, the vitamin E capsule will do just as well for hemorrhoids. I have had no personal experience in treating atrophic vaginitis.

How This Fabulous Health Vitalizer Solved Arnold V's Painful and Embarrassing Chronic Diarrhea

Arnold had been bothered by diarrhea for almost as long as he could remember. The problem was both painful and embarrassing, for he was constantly excusing himself to go to the bathroom. Since Arnold was a salesman, he was on the road a great deal of the time, and this in itself was a problem to him.

Arnold was exhausted and completely worn out by the diarrhea, so much so that he told me he barely had enough energy left to do his job. I suspected that Arnold would have a potassium deficiency, for diarrhea almost always causes one. A lack of potassium is part of the reason for a person's depleted strength and lack of energy in cases of diarrhea. A laboratory analysis of a hair sample confirmed my suspicions. I immediately asked Arnold to take some potassium gluconate tablets to correct this deficiency, but that, of course, did not solve the basic problem of the diarrhea.

For that I asked Arnold to eat yogurt 3 times a day and to take 2 *lactobacillus acidophilus* capsules after each meal. From my own past personal experience I knew this was the best possible treatment for severe diarrhea. I myself had contracted a case of "Montezuma's Revenge" many years before during a trip to Mexico. Despite everything I did, the diarrhea persisted long after I was back in my office.

At that time, I was not yet into vitamins, minerals, natural foods, and other catalytic health vitalizers as remedies for illness. One of my patients learned of my problem and told me how she had solved diarrhea for her own family.

"I have 2 daughters," Penny said, "and whenever one of them picks up a case of diarrhea, I feed her yogurt, morning, noon, and night. It takes only a day or so to clear it up. I used to try and give them lactobacillus acidophilus capsules, but they were too hard for the children to swallow. I found that yogurt works just as well. I usually add fruit of some kind to make it more appetizing for them."

As I think you know by now, I've never been averse to learning something new from my patients; so I immediately tried Penny's diarrhea remedy for myself. I used both yogurt and acidophilus capsules. Her method worked like a charm, and I was over my problem in less than a week. I've used it ever since then with great success on any patient suffering with diarrhea.

Arnold was no exception to the rule. He, too, recovered in only a few short days. His intestinal flora was restored to normal, and he quickly regained his lost strength and energy. I also had Arnold take a multi-vitamin, multi-mineral supplement, for the diarrhea had badly depleted his vitamin and mineral reserves. I'll explain that problem more fully a bit later.

Arnold still eats yogurt daily and takes the acidophilus capsules as a precautionary measure, especially when he is on the road, because of the necessity to eat in restaurants and drink strange water all the time. So far, he's had no return of his former problem.

How This Marvelous Catalytic
Health Vitalizer Can Help You

I know of no disease that can strike you down so quickly and make you feel more miserable and weak than common diarrhea. Any number of things can cause diarrhea, but they all cause destruction of the intestinal flora which must be restored before the diarrhea can be stopped. That's why yogurt and lactobacillus acidophilus capsules are so effective—they do just that.

Diarrhea is not a simple condition to be laughed at. Chronic diarrhea, especially in babies and young children, can be very serious, and here are some of the reasons why:

1. The body becomes weakened. Important food nutrients are lost. Blood sugar drops, causing hypoglycemia and further weakening, exhaustion, and fatigue.

2. Vitamins are lost, especially the oil-soluble ones, A, D, E, and K, for there is no time for them to be absorbed from the digestive tract.

3. Body fluids are washed out of the system, leading to dehydration, an extremely serious problem, especially in infants. The loss of water carries out the water-soluble vitamins, B and C.

4. Chronic diarrhea quickly depletes the body's mineral reserves, speedily causing still further problems, such as:

   a. Loss of iron which can lead to anemia.

   b. Loss of calcium. This can cause softer bones and teeth as well as nerve irritation with muscle twitching and palpitation of the heart.

   c. Loss of magnesium. This also causes innumerable nervous and muscular problems.

d. Sodium is also carried out of the body. This especially causes the weary, worn out, and dragged-down feeling that is so similar to heat exhaustion.

e. Potassium is eliminated. This is one of the most serious mineral deficiencies. Potassium is necessary for proper muscle contraction everywhere in the body. Its loss is one of the primary reasons for the loss of voluntary bowel control in diarrhea.

As you can see, then, it will be necessary for you to restore the body's vitamin and mineral reserves with vitamin and mineral supplementation while at the same times topping the diarrhea with yogurt and lactobacillus capsules.

What You Can Do for Diarrhea in Infants

If you have a baby who contracts diarrhea but who is still too small for the previous remedies I have mentioned, you can use *carob powder.* Carob tastes like expensive Dutch chocolate and can be mixed with either hot water or milk. Carob powder can be purchased at any health food store. Let me give you a case history to demonstrate its effectiveness as a catalytic health vitalizer in children.

How Fay's Severe Diarrhea Was Stopped in Only One Day. Opal M. brought her 8 month old daughter, Fay, to me for help. Fay had picked up an intestinal infection that caused a severe diarrhea. Her pediatrician had first prescribed *Parepectolin.* When that did not work, he next prescribed *Lomotil.* That was not effective either.

When Opal brought Fay to me, she was almost in a state of panic. Her little daughter had lost 5 pounds in a week and was severely dehydrated. I told her to use carob powder in her daughter's cereal and also to mix it with her milk and water.

During that first day, Opal gave her baby a total of 12 teaspoons of carob in these various ways. The next day, Fay did not have a single bowel movement. On the second day, she had a very small one, and on the third day, her stool was back to normal.

Specific Catalytic Health Vitalizers
You Can Use to Prevent Diarrhea

If you travel extensively or are forced to eat in restaurants or drink water of an unknown or questionable quality, several methods can be used to keep diarrhea from happening to you in the first place.

1. *Take Apple Cider Vinegar.* Germs or bacteria cannot live in an acid medium. If you are forced to eat food where there is any question of its safety or drink water of a questionable quality, add 2 teaspoons of apple cider vinegar to a glass of water and sip it all during your meal.

2. *Use Garlic Capsules.* A missionary friend of mine and his wife traveled extensively last year in 3 Latin American countries: Colombia, Ecuador, and Panama. They did not follow the usual tourist routes, but instead traveled into the most backward and primitive sections of these countries. They ate everything put before them and drank the same water the natives drank. The only precaution they observed was to take 8 garlic capsules every day, 2 with each meal and 2 before going to bed. They never once had even the slightest sign of diarrhea.

These Health Vitalizers
Work a Miracle for Sharon B.

Although canker sores may not be considered to be a major health problem to many people, I can assure you that they are extremely important to the person who has them. Canker sores can make eating or drinking a miserable ordeal. They may not be life-threatening, but they can cause a great deal of pain and discomfort.

I stumbled onto the perfect solution for canker sores quite by accident. It so happened that several of the patients whom I had treated for diarrhea also had canker sores. When I used yogurt and lactobacillus acidophilus capsules to heal their diarrhea, their canker sores were simultaneously healed, too.

Sharon came to me specifically for the treatment of her canker sores. She'd had them for 8 months and had tried everything she could think of with no success. She was willing to do anything, and when I suggested yogurt and acidophilus, she accepted my recommendation without question. In only one week her canker sores disappeared and have never come back. Sharon says it might not be a big deal to some people, but as far as she's concerned, it's a miracle.

What You Can Do for
Occasional Indigestion or Heartburn

No matter how healthy you are, you can occasionally suffer from some stomach distress if you eat too much or if you eat the wrong food or the wrong combinations of food. I've found that stomach upsets often come from eating too much sugar—doughnuts, cookies, pie, soft drinks, whatever.

For those occasional sieges of indigestion or heartburn, I highly recommend *papaya* tablets. They are made from the luscious melon-shaped fruit that grows in clusters on the papaya tree. It grows only in the tropics where it has been valued as both food and medicine for centuries. The papaya is often called the "medicine tree," for nearly every part of it contains some medicinal properties.

Papaya tablets stimulate your digestive system and get it going again because its enzymes—papain, mylase, and prolase—help digest the proteins and starches you have eaten. Papaya tablets will work wonders for temporary digestive problems.

13

How These Catalytic Health Vitalizers Prevent the Loss of Energy That Handicaps So Many People Today

Low blood sugar is one of the major causes of excessive exhaustion and fatigue. However, it is not the only problem that causes loss of energy. There are many others, some of which I have already discussed in previous chapters—insomnia, for example.

Even our modern living and working conditions that emphasize speed and hurrying to get things done faster and faster cause stress, strain, and excessive fatigue. Many of us are victims of this "hurry syndrome," which in itself can lead to duodenal ulcers, palpitation of the heart, high blood pressure, excessive fatigue, even an eventual nervous breakdown.

What can you do to correct this situation? Slow down . . . take it easy . . . do only one thing at a time . . . live in the ever-present now, and use the catalytic health vitalizers that I'll tell you about in this chapter. Not only will you live longer, but you'll feel a lot better and enjoy it a lot more while you're doing it.

Why Sugar and Candy Are Not Good Sources of Energy

Let me clear up a common misunderstanding about energy right here before we go on. Many people believe the commercials they see and hear on TV and the radio or the advertisements they read in magazines and newspapers about sugar—usually in the form of candy—being the best source of energy. This is simply not true. An orange, an apple, or a handful of grapes will furnish energy just as quickly as a candy bar. Not only that, but fruit is a lot more wholesome, nutritious, and long lasting as a supply of energy than candy will ever be.

Sugar taken into the body in the form of candy—or any other man-made carbohydrate—causes your blood sugar to rise rapidly, and you will feel better for perhaps 20 to 30 minutes or so. But then you'll be tired again. You see, your body will not tolerate excess sugar in the blood; so it immediately sets to work to either store it in the liver as glycogen or to let it spill over into the urine.

If you have any tendency at all toward hypoglycemia, your blood sugar will then fall far too low and you'll usually feel even worse than you did before. To prevent this high-low yo-yo-like syndrome, you need a lasting supply of energy that will carry you through the whole morning until lunch and then through the afternoon until it's time to quit work for the day.

What's the best solution, then, for this lack of energy problem? How can you best build up your strength and give your body the energy it needs? You can do that by eating high-powered foods that bring that much needed energy into your body more slowly yet *continually*, so it can be sustained at peak operating efficiency for longer periods of time, just as Norma W. does, for example.

How Norma W's Energy Is Maintained at a High Level All Day Long

Norma is a legal secretary for an extremely busy law firm. She is under a great deal of pressure to meet certain specific deadlines, and, of course, her typing of legal documents and correspondence must be meticulous. All in all, she is under a great deal of strain. At the end of a busy day she used to be so exhausted that she would almost drop over right at her desk.

Norma was using coffee, cigarettes, and a candy bar to try and quiet her nerves and regain her energy during her morning and afternoon breaks, but she found herself becoming more and more fatigued, as well as being extremely nervous and jittery. More and more mistakes were showing up in her typing, and she found herself working longer and harder, yet getting less and less done.

I've always found sunflower seeds to be one of the finest sources of energy; so I recommended to Norma that she eat them during her breaks and any time at her desk, whenever she felt even the slightest hunger pang or the least bit of sag in her energy levels. I also suggested that she substitute orange juice or apple juice for her coffee during the morning and afternoon breaks.

The last time Norma was in for her check-up, she told me that sunflower seeds had solved her energy problem in only a few days. She now feels fine, is no longer nervous and jumpy, and finds that her energy reserves are not depleted at the end of the day as they were before. Norma told me her boss was curious about her sunflower seeds and so started eating them himself— and with good results, too. He has felt an increase in his own energy levels and finds that he is able to do much more with far less effort than before.

Norma also realized a couple of side benefits that she said had to be due to the sunflower seeds, for she had made no other changes in her diet. She used to have soft nails that broke very easily. This was a nuisance to her since she spent so many of her working hours at the typewriter. About 2 weeks after she started

193

eating sunflower seeds, her nails became stronger; they stopped breaking and have stayed that way ever since.

One other benefit that both of us found hard to credit to sunflower seeds was this: Norma had been troubled with dandruff ever since she'd been a child. She'd tried everything imaginable for it, but nothing had ever helped. Even a prescription shampoo from her doctor failed to get rid of it for her.

She brushed her hair constantly to keep the dandruff down to a minimum, but it had always been troublesome to her. As Norma told me, she never wore a dark dress or sweater so the dandruff would never be seen on her shoulders. Even so, she was constantly brushing off her shoulders just to make sure they were clean.

About a month after she started on sunflower seeds, her dandruff disappeared completely, and her hair was in better condition than it had ever been. Before it had been dry and lifeless; now it looked healthy and had a beautiful appearance. As I say, she and I were both hard put to credit sunflower seeds for this miracle, but since it was the only change she had made in her diet, we had no other alternative. Sunflower seeds had to be responsible.

How This Catalytic Health Vitalizer Can Improve Your Health

Sunflower seeds may not get rid of dandruff for you, but I know for sure that they'll raise your energy levels and make you feel a lot better. Most seeds are excellent sources of many nutrients, for they are *whole foods*, but sunflower seeds are the best of all.

If you feel your energy sagging, don't reach for a candy bar; reach for the sunflower seeds instead. They won't rot your teeth or upset your stomach as the sugar and chocolate in a candy bar will. Instead, they'll raise your blood sugar naturally through their high protein content.

Additionally, they contain nearly all the minerals the body needs: phosphorus, iron, calcium, iodine, magnesium, potassium, manganese, copper, zinc, and sodium. Vitamin-wise, they have A, the B complex, and E. They also contain a huge amount of vitamin F, an important sexual stimulant that I'll discuss in more detail in the next chapter.

Athletes have found sunflower seeds to be high in energy. Some major league baseball players have taken to munching sunflower seeds in the dugout instead of chewing tobacco. People have thought for years that one extremely famous outfielder had a big cud of tobacco in his bulging left cheek. Instead, that bulge was due to sunflower seeds. Another major leaguer, a pitcher who's been around almost since the beginning of the game, it seems, credits sunflower seeds and sunflower seed oil for his good health and longevity as a player.

Russian athletes are also avid users of sunflower seeds. So is the Russian army. Every soldier carries a 2 pound bag of sunflower seeds as a survival ration. If no other food is available, he can live for several days on these seeds alone. The only other thing he needs to survive is water.

How I Restored Willard L's Sagging Energy Levels with This Wonderful Catalytic Health Vitalizer

As valuable as sunflower seeds are, and even though I do recommend them highly as an energy supplement for every patient suffering with excessive fatigue and exhaustion, they are not always the total answer. Sometimes, other catalytic health vitalizers are needed as well.

Willard came to me because he was so worn out all the time that he just couldn't seem to keep up with his job. In fact, he was afraid that he was going to lose it. "Doc, I'm so worn out all the time I can't even think straight," Willard said. "I find myself constantly doing my work over and over again because of dumb mistakes because I'm so tired my mind just seems to go blank on me. I have no zip, no zest, no sparkle, no nothing. Man, do I ever need help!"

My physical examination of Willard revealed no abnormalities that could be causing his loss of energy. A mineral analysis of a hair sample conducted by the Parmae Laboratories also proved to be negative. But when I made a comprehensive nutrient analysis of Willard's daily diet, I found him to be extremely deficient in his intake of vitamin E.

I placed Willard on 1,200 units of vitamin E each day, and in only a week he was functioning normally again. Why? Because the vitamin E he was missing helped his body use oxygen more efficiently and at the same time reduced his body's oxygen requirements.

How Vitamin E Can Help
Your Athletic Performance

No matter what sport you like to participate in, golf, tennis, bowling, swimming, jogging, walking or whatever, vitamin E can improve your performance and increase your stamina. And I think it should almost go without saying that if vitamin E can increase your physical stamina and energy levels and improve your performance, it can improve your job performance as well. But let me tell you here how much it has improved the athletic abilities of professional teams.

Even as far back as 1973, some professional athletes had come to realize how much vitamin E could do for them. The magazine, Hockey Illustrated, reported in its May 1973 issue that "The Chicago Black Hawks Are Hooked on Vitamin E." The Detroit Red Wings was another hockey team that also found that vitamin E improved athletic stamina and performance.

The Russians have reported that vitamin E supplementation improved the time of their cross-country skiers and cyclists. In fact, the reported indicated that they could estimate quite accurately the exact amount needed for various kinds of athletic events. Since that report was made, Russian athletes have dominated most of the international sports scene.

Swimming is another sport where performance can be improved by the use of vitamin E to increase stamina and energy levels. Some swimming teams have reported the success achieved in improving athletic performance with the use of megadoses of vitamin E.

A friend of mine, Ted S., goes to Colorado to ski each winter. When he first started going there, he had difficulty breathing in the high mountain altitudes of Colorado with its thin air, especially after being used to the thick humid air of Florida.

I suggested to Ted that he take 1,600 units of vitamin E daily on his next Colorado skiing trip. He found he could then breathe without any shortness of breath at all. In fact, Ted told me later that he was about the only one there who did not suffer from lack of oxygen in that rarefied air. Even natives of that state had more trouble breathing than Ted did.

As you may know, dog racing is a popular sport in Florida. One kennel owner tells me vitamin E has improved the physical abilities of several of his dogs so much that they have continued racing long beyond their normal anticipated usefulness for the sport. For those who say that improvement from taking vitamin E is imaginary or psychological, I wonder how they would explain this improvement to the greyhounds?

How Darlene T. Solved Her
Low Blood Sugar and Loss of Energy Problem

Although the best way to combat low blood sugar is to avoid refined white sugar and bleached white flour in all its forms, eating high protein foods instead, some people have found that certain high power foods also help them immensely.

For Darlene this high power food was brewer's yeast. She had suffered with all the symptoms of low blood sugar for nearly 20 years—headaches, nervousness, irritability, muscle weakness—until she discovered she could solve her problem by watching her diet. But brewer's yeast put the finishing touches on as far as Darlene was concerned; it was the icing on the cake.

I cannot argue with her, for I know that brewer's yeast is one of the best energy foods you can use. It is packed chock-full of energy building vitamins and minerals. If you will recall, I discussed it quite thoroughly back in Chapter 3. What I want to point out here is that if you do have a problem with low blood sugar and a resultant loss of energy, the proper diet and brewer's yeast could solve the problem for you just as quickly and easily as it did for Darlene.

How to Tell if You Have Low Blood Sugar

Do you suffer from depression, insomnia, anxiety, irritability, inability to concentrate, crying spells, forgetfulness, confusion, anti-social behavior? Do you often have headaches, dizziness, trembling, numbness, blurred vision, staggering, fainting or blackouts, muscular twitching? Are you troubled with exhaustion, excessive fatigue, bloating, stomach cramps, colitis, muscle and joint pains? Have you gone to your doctor time after time looking for help only to be told, "There's nothing physically wrong with you . . . it's all in your mind; you're just imagining things . . . you're neurotic . . . you'll just have to learn to live with it"?

Well, I can assure you that there's no doubt that there's something wrong if you have any of these symptoms. Chances are 99 out of 100 that you have low blood sugar. *One in every 10 people has.* In fact, without even seeing you or talking with you, I can tell you this:

If you have at least 3 of the following symptoms, it's almost a dead-sure cinch that you have hypoglycemia.

1. Chronic fatigue
2. Chronic nervous exhaustion
3. Afternoon headaches
4. Need to eat often, hunger pangs, feeling faint
5. Feeling weak and faint if meals are delayed
6. Fatigue that is relieved by food rather than rest
7. Getting shaky and weak when hungry
8. Excessive sleepiness after meals

9. Napping a lot during the day
10. Lack of energy and vitality
11. Often depressed for no reason at all

What Causes Low Blood Sugar or Hypoglycemia

I know it sounds like a physiological paradox, but a high sugar intake can result in low blood sugar. You see, the normal body keeps its blood sugar at a nearly constant level. But when a person's carbohydrate metabolism is not working properly, when it has been damaged or thrown out of whack by the constant and excessive consumption of man-made carbohydrates, then the blood sugar fluctuates up and down abnormally. The ingested sugar is absorbed so rapidly into the blood stream that the blood sugar rises far above its normal limits.

Under normal circumstances, the pancreas would secrete just enough insulin to bring the blood sugar down to its proper level. Unfortunately, over a period of time, due to the constant and heavy consumption of man-made foods containing refined white sugar and bleached white flour—for example, white bread, rolls, doughnuts, cake, cookies, ice cream, candy, soft drinks, and so on—the pancreas actually becomes trigger-happy. It secretes far too much insulin even at the slightest hint of excess sugar in the blood.

When too much insulin enters the blood stream at one time, it metabolizes too much blood sugar. Blood sugar levels then fall rapidly below normal limits. A person with hypoglycemia will then experience a wide range of symptoms that I've already mentioned. Usually, the initial symptoms will be a feeling of exhaustion and fatigue, a clammy cold skin, and sweating.

Too often people with hypoglycemia think more sugar is the answer to their problem since they usually feel better, *but only temporarily, for 20 or 30 minutes or so,* after eating sweets or consuming alcohol. But this is not true. More sugar is not the answer to the problem of hypoglycemia. The only cure for low blood sugar and its associated symptoms is not more sugar, but actually less sugar in the diet.

What You Can Do for Low Blood Sugar on Your Own

If you had a severe case of diabetes that could not be controlled by diet alone, your doctor would place you on insulin to control your blood sugar levels. However, with hypoglycemia, there is no drug or medicine to help control your blood sugar levels. Diet is the only answer. Here's what you can do for yourself.

First of all, eliminate all refined white sugar and man-made carbohydrates containing it from your daily diet. Read the labels on all canned and packaged foods to see if sugar has been added; 99 times out of 100 it has been. Even canned soups and most frozen vegetables contain sugar.

You do not need one ounce of refined white sugar to provide your body with energy. Don't let the sugar industry's advertising mislead you. Refined white sugar furnishes you only with empty calories—nothing more. It has no vitamins, no minerals, no enzymes, and absolutely no food value of any sort.

Natural carbohydrates in fresh fruits and vegetables will furnish all the energy your body needs. If you have a sweet tooth, you can always use honey as a natural sweetener. But be wise here, too. Although honey is a natural sugar with vitamins, minerals, and enzymes, you should use it sparingly if you are prone to having low blood sugar.

I have for years now satisfied my own sweet tooth with a tangerine or an apple along with a piece of extra sharp cheddar cheese for dessert. I have found that combination to be much more satisfying than a piece of cake or pie alamode.

You should eat plenty of protein in the form of fresh meat, fish, poultry, milk, eggs, and cheese. It is always best to avoid meats that have been processed with sodium nitrate and sodium nitrite. These are potent cancer causing chemicals. In fact, one scientist has found that bacon is the most dangerous food in the supermarket.

Eat lots of fresh fruits and vegetables, raw if possible. These will give you the natural carbohydrates you need for energy as well as vitamins, minerals, enzymes, cellulose, and fiber. Use stone-ground 100 percent whole wheat bread in place of white bread and whole grain cereals instead of the sugar coated ones you see advertised on television on Saturday mornings.

To increase your energy, take a high potency vitamin B supplement at least twice a day along with some desiccated liver and brewer's yeast. Large doses of vitamin B not only help to increase your energy reserves, but they also help stabilize your blood sugar levels. If you are still troubled with excessive fatigue, then take some wheat germ oil as well.

If You Take Drugs for High Blood Pressure, You Need This Catalytic Health Vitalizer, Just As Gladys F. Did

I have a great many hypertensive patients who are using a prescription drug of one sort or another to help control their blood pressure. Many of them come to me because of excessive fatigue or because of some other problem rather than hypertension.

For example, Gladys F. came to me for treatment of excessive muscular weakness and fatigue and nervous exhaustion along with a loss of mental alertness. She felt a chiropractor could help her with these problems with natural healing methods. Besides, she did not want to take any more drugs, fearing there might be some sort of a conflict or reaction with her hypertensive medication.

I found that Gladys was extremely deficient in potassium, as so often happens in patients taking medication for high blood pressure. You see, most drugs used for hypertension severely deplete the body's potassium supply.

I did not ask Gladys to discontinue her high blood pressure medication. Only the doctor who prescribed that drug for her had the right to do that. Instead, I asked Gladys to take a potassium gluconate supplement each day and to eat plenty of oranges, bananas, and fresh green vegetables to get more potassium in its natural state.

In only a few days, Gladys found that she no longer suffered from her muscular weakness and fatigue. Her nervous exhaustion disappeared, and she found she was now mentally alert and able to concentrate. She soon recovered her lost energy and has had no more trouble since then.

How You Can Recognize a Potassium Deficiency

If you are taking medicine for high blood pressure, you can suspect a potassium deficiency if you seem forgetful and absentminded or if you suffer from muscular weakness and fatigue. The earliest symptoms of a potassium deficiency are often muscular weakness and mental confusion. Other symptoms of a lack of potassium are these:

1. Itching skin
2. Soreness in the joints
3. Low resistance to colds and infections
4. More sensitivity to temperature changes; cold weather cannot be tolerated as well as before
5. Legs cramp, especially at night
6. Difficulty in relaxing and feeling at ease with others

Other Catalytic Health Vitalizers That Can Be Used for Quick Energy

Besides sunflower seeds, brewer's yeast, the vitamin B complex, vitamin E, and potassium gluconate, the following catalytic health vitalizers have been found to be of great value in restoring stamina and building energy levels:

1. *Grapes.* Grapes provide positive energy, for their sugar content is much like the blood sugar in your body. It can be

absorbed and assimilated quickly. If you lack energy, eat a half pound or more of grapes. You'll be amazed at the quick surge of energy that courses through your body.

2. *Blackstrap Molasses*. This has long been known as a food that can be used almost like a medicine, for blackstrap molasses contains organic iron and will quickly energize the weak run-down person. Patients of mine with a tired draggy feeling have reported quick energy increases after taking blackstrap molasses for breakfast.

3. *Honey*. I mentioned honey before as a natural sweetener for your sweet tooth. It will also provide a quick surge of energy in weak persons. Athletes have used it successfully, for it not only provides quick energy, but also acts as a long-lasting source of extra power.

4. *Liver*. Liver provides protein, vitamins, minerals, enzymes, and energy. Many doctors consider it as absolutely necessary for regaining health and energy in sick and weak persons. If you add liver to your diet, you'll note an improvement in a few days that will last.

If you can't stand liver, then take desiccated liver tablets. They, too, are a powerhouse of energy-building nutrients and have been used successfully by athletes for years.

5. *Wheat Germ*. A grain of wheat, like all seeds, contains all the nutriment needed for germination and growth. It contains protein, minerals, B vitamins, fats and carbohydrates, all in the correct proportions. Wheat germ has been found to be invaluable in building energy and reducing fatigue. Both wheat germ and wheat germ oil, once opened, must be refrigerated to prevent rancidity.

14

How Catalytic Health Vitalizers
Will Make You Healthier
and Much More Attractive

Not all my patients who come to me are really sick in the true sense of the word. They have no specific ailment as such to treat. They come to me because they have heard of my reputation as a doctor who uses preventive methods to help a person improve his general health so he can keep from getting sick. Although these people feel good, they want to feel even better. They want to protect their health. And without a single exception, when they follow my simple catalytic health vitalizing program, they do. I know that you can, too.

In this chapter, then, I want to give you some tips on how to better your general overall health and become more attractive by improving your external appearance. For example, you'll learn the methods my patients used to gain a healthier skin and a more attractive complexion, how they gained more beautiful hair and eyes, how they revitalized their sex lives, how they got rid of those extra inches around their waists, and how they increased their zip, their pep, and energy.

No doubt about it, when all your vital organs are healthy and functioning properly, you will feel good and you'll look good. When you're full of energy and vitality, pep and go-power, you radiate and glow all over. You literally bubble with optimistic joy and enthusiasm. And people can tell. Your personality will be positive and outgoing. This makes you attractive to everyone.

Most of the recommendations and health tips in this chapter come from my own personal, long experience in the health field. However, some of the information is based on home remedies that have been used successfully by my patients.

How to Look Better and Feel Better
No Matter How Healthy You Are Now

A few years ago I was visited by a patient who was not really sick at all. Beth H. was just under 50 years of age, and she had become deeply concerned about her future physical appearance, for as she looked around at some of her friends, she noticed how their appearances had begun to deteriorate rapidly after they turned 50, some even before. Their hair began to look dry and lifeless; deep wrinkles could be seen in their faces; many complexions were so pasty and sallow that no cosmetics could hide the unhealthy pallor; eyes were sunken and dull; fingernails had become snagged and broken; most of them had developed that unattractive middle-aged potbelly.

Although she was in good health and athletically active, Beth had never made any extra special efforts to take care of herself or maintain her good health. It just came naturally to her. But she felt that she just might be on the edge of these things happening to her, and she wanted none of it. That's why she came to me.

My physical examination of Beth revealed nothing of any great consequence. Other than being about 8 to 10 pounds overweight, there seemed to be nothing physically wrong with her. However, there was no question in my mind but that her general health could be improved. I have never yet met a person who would not feel better and look better by following my diet of natural foods and catalytic health vitalizers no matter how healthy he might be when he came to see me.

So I placed Beth on my recommended diet of fresh fruits and vegetables, 100 percent whole wheat bread, whole grain cereals, fresh meat, fish, poultry, and cheese. This diet is discussed in complete detail in Chapter 14 (Outstanding Methods I Use to Keep My Patients Well After They Get Well) of my book, *Extraordinary Healing Secrets from a Doctor's Private Files.** Unfortunately, I do not have the space to cover it fully here.

I also asked Beth not to use refined white sugar, bleached white flour or any foods containing them, and to avoid all packaged and processed man-made foods as much as possible. One of the best rules of thumb you can follow to avoid artificial or man-made foods containing chemical additives and preservatives is to *eat foods that are born—not made.*

Catalytic Health Vitalizing Vitamins and Minerals I Asked Beth to Take

Besides following my diet of natural foods and avoiding all those artificial man-made carbohydrates, I also asked Beth to take the following catalytic health vitalizing vitamins and minerals each day to help her improve her already good health:

Vitamin A	25,000 units
Vitamin D	800 units
Vitamin E	1,200 units
Vitamin C	3,000 milligrams

---

*James K. Van Fleet, *Extraordinary Healing Secrets from a Doctor's Private Files* (West Nyack, New York, 10994: Parker Publishing Company), 1977.

Vitamin B Complex

A good vitamin B supplement should furnish the following each day:

Vitamin B-1 (Thiamin)	100–300 milligrams
Vitamin B-2 (Riboflavin)	60–180 milligrams
Vitamin B-3 (Niacin)	100–300 milligrams
Vitamin B-6 (Pyridoxine)	100–300 milligrams
Vitamin B-12	100–300 micrograms
Folic Acid	100–300 micrograms
Pantothenic Acid	100–300 milligrams
Biotin	100–300 micrograms
PABA	100–300 milligrams
Calcium	2,000 milligrams (4,000 to 5,000 if elderly or poorly absorbed)
Magnesium	In proportion with calcium in dolomite
Zinc	30 milligrams

Additional supplements I asked Beth to take are these: *desiccated liver* tablets and *brewer's yeast* (these are potent sources of the B complex and fill any gaps that might be left, and they are also a valuable source of protein); *Multimineral* tablets to supply iron, iodine, copper, potassium, manganese, and phosphorus; *sea kelp* to supply trace minerals; *lecithin* for nervous stability and cholesterol control—all these as recommended by the individual manufacturer.

Now then. What were the results in Beth's case? Let me tell you exactly what she told me. After only 2 months of this regimen, Beth said her nerves were better; she had a brighter and happier disposition; she felt more energetic and full of life; her complexion had improved and was even more clear than before; her digestion was better; and her bowel movements were much easier. Beth also lost 8 unwanted pounds. She said that the improvement in her general health was amazing to her, especially since she hadn't really felt sick in the first place.

See why I say I know that if you follow the same program that Beth did you'll look better and feel better no matter how healthy you are right now? Beth is only one example. I could give you dozens of others.

Environmental Factors That Increase Vitamin and Mineral Requirements

If you still feel you don't need vitamin and mineral supplements, let me give you some information that could change your mind. Do you take either prescription or over-the-counter drugs? (Aspirin counts, too.) If you do, I know you need extra vitamins and minerals, and here's why: Prescription and over-the-counter drugs along with many other factors in our environment destroy the vitamins we take into our bodies. For example, if you take an antacid preparation for gastric distress or heartburn, it will destroy vitamin B-1 because of the alkaline medium it provides. Mineral oil dissolves and destroys all the fat-soluble vitamins A, D, E, and K. Barbiturates and anti-convulsant drugs destroy folic acid of the B complex. Sulfa drugs cause troublesome digestive upsets by destroying your friendly intestinal flora. Neomycin interferes with the absorption of vitamins A and B-12.

Here's a list of more of the environmental factors that destroy catalytic health vitalizers and increase your vitamin and mineral requirements:

1. Drinking alcohol, coffee, or tea destroys vitamins A and all of the B complex.
2. Smoking tobacco or marijuana destroys B-1, B-2, B-6, B-12, folic acid, and vitamin C.
3. Taking birth control pills destroys vitamins in the B complex and vitamin E.
4. Sleeping pills destroy the vitamins of the B complex.
5. Mental or physical stress and strain destroy vitamins of the B complex and vitamins C and P.

6. Excessive ingestion of sugared products such as candy, cookies, soft drinks, and so on, destroys vitamins of the B complex, especially B-1, B-3, and choline.

7. Eating raw clams destroys vitamin B-1.

8. Exposure to radiation destroys B-6 and F (the sex vitamin).

9. Exposure to chlorine (as in swimming pools and drinking water) destroys vitamin E.

10. Eating rancid fat or rancid oil destroys vitamins E and K.

11. Taking aspirin destroys vitamins C, K, and P.

I'm sure you can see from this that practically everyone needs supplemental vitamins and minerals. This is only one of the reasons I have no patience at all with doctors who say you don't need to take vitamins and minerals.

I know that doctors who say that vitamin and mineral supplements won't cure disease or help a patient to feel better or look better have never used them in their practices. Had they done so, they would know how valuable these catalytic health vitalizers can be in restoring or maintaining a person's good health.

**How You Can Have More Attractive
Skin and a Gorgeous Complexion**

A variety of catalytic health vitalizers is necessary to maintain your skin in a good state of health. If your skin is dry, rough, scaly, and easily infected, if you have problems with blackheads, pimples, and pus formations, if you have a dry scalp with coarse hair and dandruff, you no doubt need more of the catalytic health energizer, vitamin A. Twenty-five to 30,000 units a day should clear up this problem for you.

Don't worry about getting too much vitamin A if you stay in this dosage range. Vitamin A can be toxic, but only if you take 100,000 units every day for *many, many months*. No fatalities have ever been reported from an overdosage of vitamin A.

The absence of the catalytic health vitalizer, the vitamin B complex, can also cause problems such as a dry, rough, cracked skin, and dull dry hair. To determine which vitamin is lacking, either A or the B complex, you must know the other symptoms of their deficiencies.

If you are deficient in vitamin A, you will also be troubled with night blindness, bright lights will bother you, and you'll have an increased susceptibility to infections. Other symptoms of a vitamin B deficiency are excessive fatigue, poor appetite, nervousness, and gastrointestinal disorders. If you are not sure which deficiency, A or B, is causing your problems, then take both of them. I have had some patients solve their skin problems with vitamin A, others with vitamin B, while still others required a combination of the 2 catalytic health vitalizers.

For instance, one of my patients, Paula E., had the worst acne problem I have ever seen. She required large amounts of vitamin A internally to clear up the condition, along with vitamin E oil externally to heal the scarred facial tissues.

However, Grace N. had a large-pored oily complexion with lots of acne. When I gave her the B complex, desiccated liver, and brewer's yeast, her acne cleared up and her complexion became satiny smooth and beautiful.

Why Charlotte Has a Perfect Complexion

Another patient of mine, Charlotte L., is 79 years old. She is one of the most amazing people I have ever met. She is in excellent health. Her face doesn't have a single wrinkle in it; her skin is smooth, soft, and beautiful. How does she manage that? Well, she doesn't smoke and she doesn't get too much sun on her face, both of which can cause premature facial wrinkles. She avoids refined white sugar and bleached white flour. She also takes all the catalytic health vitalizers that I recommend for her. However, she does 2 more things on her own which she says add the finishing touches, to give her a perfect complexion.

For years now Charlotte has been using a brewer's yeast face mask and vitamin E skin cream each night before going to bed. She mixes some powdered brewer's yeast in sterile water and applies the mixture to her face. She lets this dry and leaves it on for about 10 minutes. Then she washes it off and applies a vitamin E vanishing cream to her face and massages it in.

Charlotte says the brewer's yeast cleanses her pores and tightens her skin, while the vitamin E skin cream helps to keep her complexion soft, smooth, and supple. I certainly cannot disagree with her method, for her face is radiantly young. It is living proof that what she is doing is the right thing to do.

Zinc Is Also a Marvelous Catalytic Health Vitalizer for the Skin

I have used zinc in case after case of acne and eczema where nothing else would help. Thirty milligrams a day is all that is required in most instances.

For example, Olivia J. had been troubled with acne since she was 13 years old. It got worse for her over the years despite a variety of creams and lotions that she used. She was 22 when she came to see me. Thirty milligrams of zinc gluconate daily cleared up her complexion completely in only a month.

Owen D. had suffered with acne for nearly 4 years. He, too, was deficient in zinc. After only 2 weeks of taking 30 milligrams of zinc gluconate daily his face became clear and smooth. All his friends were amazed at the change.

Zinc has also helped some patients who suffered with troublesome body odor. I don't understand the physiology of this at all, but I do know it has obtained results. Philip N., for instance, had long been troubled with underarm perspiration and odor along with badly sweating feet. A month after his taking 30 milligrams of zinc gluconate daily, his body odor vanished and his feet stayed dry all day long.

Zinc has resolved scalp odor and dandruff for some of my patients with this problem. Scott K. had always been plagued with a dandruff condition. His scalp would itch and begin to flake about 3 days after washing his hair. After I placed him on 30 milligrams of zinc each day, this problem stopped altogether. He is no longer bothered by dandruff or an itching scalp even if he goes a week or more without shampooing his hair.

How Vitamin E Oil Can Help Your Complexion

If you have some acne scars, you can use vitamin E oil or vitamin E cream externally and take 1,200 units of vitamin E orally each day. This procedure will either remove these scars or make them less noticeable over a period of time. Much patience is required; so you must be persistent with this treatment. Vitamin E oil or cream is extremely useful for crows feet around the eyes and for preventing or reducing the wrinkles caused by the aging process.

How to Make Your Eyes Sparkle and Shine

Your eyes are dependent upon good nutrition for their luster, brightness, and beauty. The following catalytic health vitalizers are absolutely necessary if you want to have good eyesight and more attractive eyes.

1. Vitamin A is a specific for the healthy eye. In 119 cases of conjunctivitis among school children, a vitamin deficiency was discovered in all of them. Another condition caused by a lack of vitamin A is xerosis, a disorder in which the eyeball loses its luster and becomes dry and lifeless in appearance.

2. A lack of the B complex will cause inflammation of the eyelids and loss of eyelashes. The eyelids may smart and itch; the eyes may grow tired and red; and vision may be poor and unable to be improved by glasses.

3. If vitamin C is missing, the eyes do not get enough oxygen. As a result, the capillaries will enlarge and the eyes will become red. To use an over-the-counter medication to "get the red out" only makes the situation worse. Vitamin C is the correct answer to this problem.

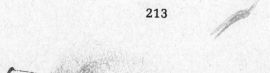

4. A lack of vitamin D will cause cataracts. In animal experiments in the laboratory, a deficiency of D caused cloudy lenses and poor vision.

How a Smile Can Improve Your Good Looks

For a winning smile, use lots of calcium in the form of dolomite to anchor those teeth to the jawbone; and along with it, use lots of vitamin C to keep the gum tissues in good condition. One of my former patients, who is now a student at the University of Florida, wrote me the following letter:

> I was offered a free tooth inspection and cleaning at the dental hygienist school here. Naturally I accepted. When I told the girl I hadn't been to a dentist for more than 2 years she could hardly believe it. She even called her teacher, a dentist, over to see my teeth.
>
> They were both surprised because I had no signs of any cavities and hardly any plaque. I attribute my good dental health to your program of fresh fruits and vegetables, vitamin and mineral supplements. Before I came to your office, Doctor, I used to get a couple of cavities every year and I also had a lot of gum problems. Since I stopped eating junk foods, I've never had a cavity and my gums are in a lot better shape, too.

How to Avoid the Potbelly of Middle Age

You can avoid the potbelly of middle age primarily by not eating man-made foods that contain refined white sugar or bleached white flour. These are artificial carbohydrates that stick to your body like glue and shoot your weight up like a rocket.

Instead of these foods, make your diet consist primarily of fresh fruits and fresh vegetables. I do not mean that you should become a vegetarian. You should get plenty of protein in the form of meat, fish, poultry, cheese, milk, and so on, but *raw fruits and vegetables are the secret to a lean body and a vigorous, healthy long life.*

If you can eat the fruit or vegetable either raw or cooked, *eat it raw.* Raw fruits and vegetables are rich in vitamins, minerals, and enzymes. They nourish the eyes and skin with vitamins A and C. Raw foods enrich the bloodstream with iron, copper, calcium, and phosphorus. They are a powerful source of natural energy to your body.

Raw foods improve the appetite and do wonders for the digestive system. They put a rein on the urge for excessive seasoning. Raw fruits and vegetables provide bulk and cellulose, stimulate the muscular walls of the intestine, and provide healthful regularity without harmful laxatives. To sum it up, raw foods not only make you feel better; they also make you look better.

As Dan M. told me, "I've had no more problem with my bowel movements since going on your raw fruit and vegetable diet, Doc. And since I've stopped eating all those man-made carbohydrates you warned me about, I've lost 12 pounds without any effort whatever. My energy levels have really gone up, and I feel terrific now."

If you do happen to have a severe overweight problem, say 20 pounds or more, then I would highly recommend that you get a copy of my extremely helpful book, *Doctor Van Fleet's Amazing New "Non-Glue Food" Diet.* * This book has shown hundreds of people how to lose weight quickly, easily, and permanently.

How You Can Revitalize Your Sex Life

Sexual problems do not normally bring patients to my office; they usually come for other reasons. However, in the process of taking their case histories, I often find that many of the older ones have given up sexual relations with their partners. They think they're "over the hill" and that nothing can be done about it.

---

*James K. Van Fleet, *Doctor Van Fleet's Amazing New "Non-Glue-Food" Diet* (West Nyack, New York, 10994: Parker Publishing Company), 1974.

Take Tom G., for instance. He was in his early sixties. He told me he had sexual intercourse with his wife only once a month, if then. She was perfectly willing and physically able, but he was impotent and incapable of making love to her except on rare occasions. Tom said his wife was sympathetic and understanding, but he knew she was frustrated and wished he were sexually more capable.

Through my years of experience, I have found that impotence is usually more dietetic than psychological, and Tom's case was no exception. His dietary analysis revealed a lack of *vitamin F*, a deficiency I have often found in older men who are impotent and incapable of satisfactory sexual intercourse. I will say, though, that a vitamin F deficiency is not confined only to older men; I've encountered men in their twenties and thirties whose vitamin F deficiency caused them to be sexually inadequate.

Actually, the essential fatty acids are not vitamins in the strictest sense of the word since they are required by the body in grams rather than milligrams for good health. These essential fatty acids, which are known as vitamin F, are absolutely essential for a normal, healthy sex drive.

They are found in sunflower, safflower, corn, cottonseed, soybean, and peanut oils. They are not found in olive oil. I had Tom take 2 tablespoons of sunflower oil (my favorite) each day—one tablespoon at breakfast, the other with supper. Within less than a month, he was enjoying normal sexual relations again with his wife at least once a week, sometimes more often.

Another Catalytic Health Vitalizer
That Is Necessary for a Normal Sex Life

I have also found a deficiency of zinc to be responsible for impotence in all ages, not just in older men only. A lack of zinc can also be responsible for infertility in the male. Let me give you a quick example of this from my case history file.

Walter K. and his wife, Caroline, had been married for 3 years and were still childless. Both were in their mid-twenties, apparently healthy, and they wanted a child very much.

As is so often the case, Walter felt sure the problem was Caroline's fault. His male ego would not accept the fact that he might not be fertilizing the female egg with a viable male sperm. A laboratory analysis of a hair sample from Walter revealed he was badly deficient in zinc.

Now zinc is absolutely essential for normal sexual function and fertility; so I had Walter take 60 milligrams of zinc gluconate daily for one month and then reduced his intake to 30 milligrams a day. They now have 2 healthy children.

How Prescription Drugs Can Also Ruin Your Love Life

If you're taking some sort of medicine, especially one for high blood pressure, all the aphrodisiacs in the world might not do you any good. You see, one of the adverse reactions of many of the drugs used for hypertension is to render a man completely useless for making love.

One of my patients, Jack B., was taking the drug, hygroton, for hypertension. He became impotent shortly after starting his medication and asked his doctor if this could be his problem. His doctor said unequivocally that it was not.

However, after Jack posed the question to me, I checked out the drug, hygroton, in my *Physicians' Desk Reference*. This is a complete book of all the drugs used by medical doctors. It is published by Medical Economics Company, a division of Litton Industries, at Oradell, New Jersey, 07649.

Sure enough, one of the adverse reactions of the drug Jack was taking was a reduction of sexual performance and desire. When Jack pointed this out to his medical doctor, he finally was able to get the prescription changed to one not having such side effects.

One of the drugs with the worst reputation for ruining sexual performance is *Guanethidine*. It is usually prescribed under the trade name *Esimil* or *Ismelin*. Other hypertensive medications that can interfere with sexual desire or performance in some persons are *Aldomet, Entonyl,* and *Eutron.*

If you are taking any sort of drug, whether for high blood pressure, nervousness, ulcers, or whatever, and you suspect it of ruining your sex life, ask your doctor to level with you and tell you the straight truth. If he won't do that, then go to the library and look the drug up in the *Physicians' Desk Reference*. Then show your doctor your findings and see if he won't prescribe something else that will be just as effective without spoiling your sexual relationships with your partner. If he feels that your sex life isn't important and refuses to change your prescription, then change doctors. As A. P. Herbert says in his book, *Holy Deadlock*, "If the bedroom is not right, then every room in the house is wrong."

15

How You Can Use These Miracle Catalytic Health Vitalizers to Stay Younger Longer

I would first like to discuss the methods you can use to extend your prime of life. Your aim should be not only to live longer, but also to extend your prime of life—those best years—so you can be physically and mentally active, healthy, alert, and energetic right up to your last day.

As I said in the last chapter, much of my practice is based on using preventive methods to help my patients avoid disease and to eliminate health problems even before they happen. I also use these same methods to keep my patients well after they get well.

The best time, of course, to prevent these problems of older age is not when you're 65 or 70, but when you're still in your early thirties, if not before, for that's when most of these ailments actually begin. Take rheumatism or arthritis, for example. It simmers in your body for a long time like a teakettle on the back of the stove until it finally boils over to get your attention.

Then I would like to tell you about some of the methods you can use to heal these problems of older age, if they do happen to come your way. A great many of these ailments, such as prostatic enlargement, osteoporosis, high blood pressure, arthritis and rheumatism, can be minimized or eliminated altogether by proper nutrition, including such catalytic health vitalizers as vitamins, minerals, enzymes, and natural foods.

How to Extend Your "Prime of Life" 15 to 20 Years

Dr. Roger J. Williams, the renowned biochemist, research scientist, and author of many books on health and nutrition, believes that proper nutrition—including general amounts of these 2 highly important catalytic health vitalizers, vitamins C and E—can extend the healthy life span or the prime of life of people who are already middle-aged. Of course, the greatest hope for stretching out the life span exists if proper nutrition of the highest quality has been emphasized from prenatal development to old age.

Dr. Linus Pauling, a Nobel Prize winner for his work in biochemistry, feels the same way. Although Dr. Pauling realizes that medicines, drugs, and surgery all have their place, he is much more interested in preventing disease. After years of scientific research and investigation, he made the following recommendations for maintaining one's good health at a recent meeting of the International Academy of Preventive Medicine in Kansas City, Missouri.

1. A daily supplement of large amounts of vitamin C.
2. A daily supplement of liberal amounts of vitamin E.
3. An adequate intake of all other vitamins and minerals.

4. A sharp reduction in the amount of sugar consumed.

5. Avoidance or rejection of the tobacco habit.

Dr. Pauling says in effect that if a person would follow these 5 recommendations, he could increase both the length of his life and his period of health and well-being by as much as 20 years.

Let me now discuss how not only vitamins C and E but also other catalytic health vitalizers have turned back the clock for many of my patients and given them even better health than when they were younger.

How This Catalytic Health Vitalizer Increased Michael W's Zest for Life

Michael was just over 50 when he came to see me, but most people would have guessed that he was at least 10 years older. His face was tired, worn, and lined; he had no stamina, no vitality; and he was completely exhausted long before the end of his work day. While taking his case history, I asked Michael about his sex life. He laughed sarcastically and said, "What sex life?"

My physical examination of Michael, along with laboratory analyses of blood, urine, hair samples, and a dietary analysis, revealed that his intake of all vitamins and minerals, especially vitamin C, was almost nil. Michael subsisted primarily on man-made carbohydrates—processed, packaged, and canned foods—for he thoroughly disliked fruits and vegetables.

I asked Michael to change his eating habits as much as possible to natural foods. I also had him take a high potency multi-vitamin, multi-mineral supplement. Then I added massive amounts of vitamin C—10,000 milligrams per day—for a variety of reasons.

First of all, Michael needed more vitamin C because he was not eating enough fresh fruits and vegetables. Second, most of his symptoms—aching bones, joints, and muscles, excessive fatigue, weakness, shortness of breath, and finally, impotence—pointed to a major vitamin C deficiency. Third, recent scientific research indicated that this catalytic health vitalizer was increasingly needed for normal sexual activity as a person grows older.

Michael's recovery was so rapid and so complete that it was almost like watching a miracle take place. He quickly recovered his stamina, and his energy levels rose so he was no longer exhausted at the end of the day. He lost that tired, worn-out look, and his faced appeared 10 years younger than before. And last, although certainly not least, Michael's sex life became normal again. As he told me, the strained relations that had existed between him and his wife vanished as they became ardent lovers again.

What This Magnificent Catalytic Health Vitalizer Can Do for You

There is no reason for you to grow old in the biological sense if you get enough vitamin C in your diet. By that I mean there is no reason for you to suffer the ravages of old age that so many people do. Old age does not have to be synonymous with sickness, misery, and ill-health. Let me give you one example of this.

An uncle of mine, often regarded as a "health nut" by his friends, watched his food intake carefully. He ate no man-made carbohydrates whatever, avoided all processed and packaged foods, and ate fresh fruits and vegetables, most of which were grown in his own orchard and garden. He took vitamin and mineral supplements every day. As he grew older, he increased the intake of vitamin C to 10,000 milligrams every day. He also took 1,600 units of vitamin E daily.

Uncle David lived to be 96 years old and was killed while driving his own car in an automobile accident that was not his own fault. (A car pulled out in front of him from a side road onto a main highway without stopping.) When my uncle died, he had all his own teeth and his own hair. He wore glasses only to read. He appeared to be 65 or 70 rather than 96. He outlived all his younger sisters and brothers, including my own father.

This indicates that the aging process can be slowed down or

eliminated completely. I am not saying we can live forever—far from it. Die we must when our time is up, but there is no reason to die of disease and debility—only from years alone. Vitamin C is one of the biggest factors in preventing the aging process.

Vitamin C has also been found to be one of the 2 key elements (vitamin E is the other one) in the prevention of atherosclerosis, a form of hardening of the arteries with fatty degeneration of the connective tissues of the arterial walls. That old adage, "You're as old as your arteries," still holds true. It's not your actual calendar years that make you old, but the condition of your cardiovascular system.

When you have plenty of vitamin C circulating in your bloodstream, the triglycerides that form fatty deposits in the blood vessels in atherosclerosis are broken down into free fatty acids and then utilized or eliminated. Large doses of vitamin C can keep your blood vessels as clean as if they had been swept with a broom.

If you now have hardening of the arteries, start taking plenty of vitamin C. But you must be patient. The beneficial effects of taking large amounts of vitamin C will not take place overnight. It takes 5 or 6 months before the benefits can be seen. But don't wait. If you do have arteriosclerosis, time is of the essence. Clogged arteries can kill without warning.

If you have sexual problems that have not been eliminated by either vitamin F or zinc—both of which must be present in your body for normal sexual activity—then add lots of vitamin C to your regimen. This could well be the answer you've been looking for. And sex is important, no matter how old you are. If you doubt that, you ought to talk with some of the attendants in nursing homes.

So if you're aiming for a prime of life that will continue long after you're 60, if you want to keep your youthful appearance, if you want to retain the sparkle in your eyes and the elasticity in your arteries, then increase your vitamin C intake right now— while you're still in that prime of life. Unless your body cells are kept saturated with this remarkable catalytic health vitalizer, old age can sneak up on you before you know it. If you really want to be your own best friend, you'll increase your daily intake of vitamin C right now.

How This Incredible Catalytic Health Vitalizer Extended Ray C's Prime of Life

Vitamin E is the second catalytic health vitalizer that Dr. Pauling recommended be taken in liberal amounts to extend a person's prime of life.

How does vitamin E work to do this? Although not everything is known about how vitamin E functions in the body, it is known that it can delay old age and prolong the prime of life because it has strong antioxidant properties (just as vitamin C does), and this prevents harmful and unwanted oxidations in the body. It is also known by laboratory experiments with animals that a vitamin E deficiency has been observed to produce biochemical and physiological changes exactly like those that occur in old age.

However, the best proof of how well a catalytic health vitalizer works is not always scientific, but clinical; so let me tell you about Ray C's case right here.

Ray came to me for a vascular condition (venous thrombosis) more than 7 years ago. Even though I cleared up his vascular condition in less than 2 months, he has continued to take 1,600 units of vitamin E each day as a preventive method to prevent any further cardiovascular conditions from developing. At the time, neither of us gave any thought to how the vitamin E would prolong Ray's prime of life or improve his external appearance.

Just recently, Ray applied for some additional life insurance. His agent, a friend but not a patient of mine, called me the other day and said, "Jim, what in the world are you doing for Ray? He looks to me to be in better health than he was when he first came to see me for life insurance years ago. I swear he doesn't look as if he's aged a bit. In fact, if anything he looks even younger. Has he discovered the secret of eternal youth in your office? Let me in on it, Jim. Whatever it is you're doing for Ray, I want you to do the same for me, too!"

"Forrest, it's the vitamin E he's been taking," I said. "It'll add at least 10 years or even more to your prime of life for you. Come on down and see me. I'll do the same thing for you that I've done for Ray."

How This Amazing Catalytic Health Vitalizer Can Help You, Too

I don't care how old you are; if you're not taking vitamin E, then you ought to start doing so right now. It will improve the condition of your heart and blood vessels. It will help your body use oxygen more efficiently, reduce fatigue, and increase your energy. It will help prevent or reduce the wrinkles in your skin (a sure sign of aging) when you use it externally as well as taking it orally.

Dr. Denham Harman, M.D., Ph.D., of the University of Nebraska College of Medicine, is quite outspoken and optimistic about the potential benefits of adding vitamin E to the diet. "This approach offers the prospect of an increase in the average life expectancy to beyond 85 years and a significant increase in the number of people who will live to well beyond 100 years, along with accompanying increases in the period of healthy, effective living," he says.

How to Stay Younger Longer: Three Case Histories

Dr. Pauling's third recommendation was to be sure to take an adequate amount of all other vitamins and minerals. This would include vitamins A and D, the B complex, as well as the minerals calcium, potassium, magnesium, iron, and zinc. I want now to tell you about 3 of my patients who took all these catalytic health vitalizers along with liberal amounts of C and E and the results that were gained.

1. Neal B., a patient of mine for 12 years now, is 73. He appears to be no more than 55. Neal has been taking the full

complement of vitamins and minerals that I recommend if a person wants to remain healthy and stay younger longer.

In Florida, water skiing is a popular sport. However, you normally do not expect to see a man in his seventies enjoying it, but Neal does. He still goes water skiing at least once or twice every week.

He goes up stairs 2 at a time and runs a couple of miles every day. Neal does a lot of yard work and grows a large garden. He also has extensive flower beds. He never seems to tire out. In fact, Neal has more energy than many men 20 years younger.

2. Five years ago Terry L. and his wife, Eva, started on my catalytic vitalizing program of vitamins, minerals, and natural foods. Both of them would tell you it has made an unbelievable difference in their physical and mental health and well-being.

Terry is now 68 and Eva 62. They sleep well, and have had no headaches, constipation, high blood pressure, colds or flu since starting this health-building and life-prolonging program. They have just finished building a barn on their acreage. They did every bit of the work themselves except for the electrical wiring.

3. Ward D. is 85 and extremely active. He owns and runs a large nursery and citrus tree farm. He still digs up the trees for his customers himself. He lets his 50 year old son sit in the office and do all the book work. You can guess immediately which one has constipation, high blood pressure, and a weight problem.

Ward attributes his long and healthy life to natural foods, vitamin and mineral supplements, and lots of physical activity. "I don't have a rocking chair in the house," he says. "I've seen too many people retire from work to a rocking chair and rock themselves right into the grave in a couple of years."

Ward still has his own teeth. On his last trip to the dentist, he was told he had the bones of a 40 year old man. Both Ward and I give full credit to dolomite for this.

Other Factors That Will Extend Your Prime of Life

The fourth recommendation Dr. Pauling made was to sharply reduce the amount of sugar consumed. Many research scientists in the field of nutrition—for example, Doctors Dennis Burkitt, T. L. Cleave, Neal Painter, and John Yudkin, all of England—agree with Dr. Pauling on this point. So do such prominent American doctors as Roger Williams, E. Cheraskin, W. M. Ringsdorf, Jr., Alan H. Nittler, and Henry G. Bieler.

I've already talked about some of the problems sugar can cause. So rather than discuss it any further, I would simply like to sum up the adverse effects of sugar this way:

> *People in their twenties who consume large amounts of sugar have the same kind of blood vessels as people in their seventies.*

I really don't think I need say any more than that.

Dr. Pauling's fifth recommendation is to avoid or reject the tobacco habit altogether. Cigarettes cause lung cancer as well as many other diseases. Three of my closest friends have died from lung cancer directly attributable to smoking cigarettes.

However, I do not want to talk about smoking anymore here. Tons of material—books, magazine and newspaper articles, government publications, medical reports, etc.—have been written about the hazards of smoking. Frankly, I can think of nothing to add to what has already been written, if you haven't been convinced of the dangers of smoking by now.

Other Tips to Help Prolong Your Prime of Life

1. *Keep mentally alive after you retire.* Florida is a state with a great many people over the age of 60. Those who retire to that rocking chair and who live in the past soon die. Those who retire and become active in some avocation, no matter what it is, stay young. The point is, you don't have to retire from life when you retire from your job. Mental activity will keep you young.

2. *Physical activity also keeps you young.* "What you don't use, you lose," is as applicable to the muscles as to the brain. Walking, swimming, or any sort of physical activity you can participate in without placing a strain on your heart or blood vessels is good for you. I walk 5 miles every day without fail, rain

or shine. It does not tire me out, nor do I run short of breath. Walking keeps my cardiovascular and respiratory systems in excellent condition.

3. *Eat less to live longer.* You already know the kinds of food I recommend. The only thing left for me to say here is *don't eat when you're not hungry.* Don't overload your digestive system with unnecessary food or your circulatory system with unwanted pounds. Each extra pound of weight adds 200 miles of tiny blood vessels. That places an undue strain on your heart.

How to Solve the Problems of Older Age

I now want to talk about some of the problems of older age and what you can do to take care of them if they do happen to come your way. Since I've already discussed such conditions as arthritis, coronary artery thrombosis, glaucoma, prostate problems, and kidney stones previously, I'll not cover these again here even though they are usually considered to be ailments of older people.

How This Fabulous Catalytic Health Vitalizer Controlled Peter M's Intermittent Claudication

Peter had been attending his company picnic in the summer of 1972. He had been playing softball and while running the bases from home to third on a long triple, he was forced to stop halfway between second and third with severe cramps in the calves of both legs.

After a few hours, the severe pains subsided, and for a while Peter thought he was well again. However, he soon learned that this was not the case, for a few days later the severe cramps and pain returned after he walked only a couple of blocks. The doctor to whom he went diagnosed his condition as intermittent claudication and used vasodilating drugs and anticoagulants (blood-thinning drugs). However, when Peter did not improve after 3 months treatment, he came to me.

I immediately placed Peter on 1,200 units of vitamin E daily.

Within 3 weeks he was much improved, and in only 2 months he was completely symptom-free. He could walk or run again without pain. He played golf every week on a long and hilly 18 hole course without any trouble, even though he walked all the way.

He did this for 5 years and then had a mild recurrence on the golf course one day. When this happened, I increased his vitamin E intake to 1,600 units every day. This relieved his symptoms again completely. He has never had a return of his former problem with this dosage level.

Peter's case shows that vitamin E is the best possible treatment for intermittent claudication. In fact, it is a specific. When the proper amount of vitamin E is given, the pain and cramps disappear almost immediately, for the oxygen requirements of the tissues are greatly reduced.

What You Should Do if You Suffer from Intermittent Claudication

The first symptoms of intermittent claudication (the result of hardening of the arteries in the legs) seem unimportant. Usually the person will have been walking for a time—shopping, out for a stroll, even just walking back and forth on the job—when suddenly he will have to stop because of a severe painful cramp in the calf of one leg. Standing still for a short time relieves the pain. Then walking can be resumed. Eventually, both the frequency and the severity of the muscular cramps become greater and the distance the person can walk before they occur becomes shorter. In time, both legs will be affected and the person will no longer be ambulatory.

Intermittent claudication is a very serious disease. If the patient lives long enough, it will progress to gangrene and eventual amputation of one or both legs. Second, the incidence of heart attack or death from heart failure is greatly increased with intermittent claudication.

Conventional medical methods are of little use, for vasodilators and anticoagulants do not help the patient significantly. However, vitamin E does help—so much so that it can be considered as a specific therapeutic agent for intermittent claudication, thrombophlebitis, and other circulatory diseases of the lower extremities. This statement is not based only on my own findings. Let me give you some of the results that have been obtained by other doctors.

Dr. Knut Haeger, a Swedish blood vascular surgeon, and 2 English doctors, A. M. Boyd and J. Marks, found that vitamin E caused significant improvements in patients with intermittent claudication where conventional drugs had failed.

Dr. Haeger found it necessary to perform leg amputations on 10.6 percent of the patients not receiving vitamin E therapy (11 cases out of 104 patients). However, the amputation rate was only 1.1 percent (one case out of 95) in the patients receiving vitamin E treatment. Dr. Wilfrid E. Shute, a Canadian medical doctor who is an expert in vitamin E therapy, feels this amputation might not have been necessary if the patient had received vitamin E sooner.

Doctors Marks and Boyd found that the survival rate among intermittent claudication patients receiving vitamin E was far greater than for those who did not receive it. These statistics simply confirm what I have already said: *Vitamin E is a specific for intermittent claudication.*

How Osteoporosis Can Be Cured, or Better Yet, Avoided

Osteoporosis is a thinning or weakening of the bones by loss of calcium. It is a disease found primarily in older people and is caused by 2 things, namely:

1. Cortisone used for treatment of arthritis,
2. Insufficient intake of calcium.

Let's look at the first cause. Better yet, let me give you a specific example. I had a patient, Vera L., who had rheumatoid arthritis. Her previous doctor, a prominent specialist in arthritic and rheumatic diseases, used cortisone therapy to treat her. One day, after several months of this treatment, Vera bumped her arm on a chair when she lost her balance and fell. After a few days her arm still hurt so badly; so she went to her doctor. An x-ray revealed that it was broken.

When she asked her doctor why, he said, "This often happens with cortisone treatment of arthritis." Vera stopped her cortisone therapy at once and came to me.

I immediately placed her on 5,000 milligrams of calcium every day in the form of dolomite along with 800 units of vitamin E. In a short time, her bones were back to normal. Incidentally, when the other doctor removed the cast from her broken arm, he was amazed to see how well and how quickly the bone had healed.

Osteoporosis resulting from cortisone treatment leaves the bones of the body like termite infested wood. They will bear no weight and are easily broken, for there is not enough calcium in them. Arthritis specialists say it is not unusual for patients to suffer loss of 30 to 50 percent of their bone mass after several years of cortisone treatment.

Osteoporosis in older age can be prevented no matter what the cause, whether cortisone treatment or simply an insufficient calcium intake. It requires only a higher amount of calcium each day with some vitamin D to insure proper absorption and assimilation.

I use no less than 2,000 milligrams of calcium, sometimes as much as 4 to 5,000 milligrams for older patients who have suffered a broken bone. A laboratory analysis of a hair sample 30 to 60 days later shows me whether I should raise or lower the amount.

How to Prevent or Cure Another Problem of Older Age: Leukoplakia

Leukoplakia, a disease often found in older patients with an insufficient vitamin E intake, is a chronic patchy and painful hardening of any of the mucous membranes. These patches are often thought to be precancerous, and the usual medical treatment is surgical removal. However, I have found that is not always necessary, as shown in the following case history.

Doris V. developed leukoplakia of the mucous membranes of

231

the lower lip and the inside of her left cheek. Having read of Dr. Wilfrid E. Shute's success in treating leukoplakia with vitamin E, I decided to try that before referring her to a surgeon. I used 1,200 units daily, and on this dosage the leukoplakia disappeared. Then I reduced her intake to 800 units a day, but found that with this level the problem began to recur. Raising her dosage back to 1,200 units caused the leukoplakia to again disappear.

This experience gave me guidance for my next leukoplakia patient, Jeanette F. Jeanette was 78. She had developed leukoplakia inside and outside her vaginal area. Her regular doctor treated her with hormones, salves, and so on, but after a few weeks of treatment, she became worse. She then went to a specialist in geriatric diseases who was also unable to help her. He told her that her mucous membranes were dried up, but that was normal in older female patients.

When Jeanette came to me, she was in absolute misery. She could hardly bear to sit down because of the pain. I immediately placed her on 800 units of vitamin E daily, to be taken orally, and gave her some vitamin E oil (not cream) to apply locally. After a few days of this treatment she began to feel better. In a month's time she was completely free of her ailment.

How to Keep Your Mind Young and Vital

Do you find yourself forgetting things that used to be easy to remember? Do you tend to remember events of your earlier days yet forget what happened yesterday or the day before? Do you ramble in your conversation, jumping from one subject to another for no reason at all? Have your children told you you're getting old, maybe even senile? Do you think you are?

Well, I have good news for you. I can tell you right now that chances are you're not. Most cases of so-called senility are caused not by old age, but by a vitamin B complex deficiency. The symptoms of senility and a B complex deficiency are basically the same: mental confusion, forgetfulness, apathy, all of which are indicators of decreased brain activity.

So if you (or your children) think you're getting senile and ought to be packed off to the old folks' home, forget it. Take a high potency vitamin B complex, add some brewer's yeast for good measure, and I'd be willing to bet you'll be back to normal in no time at all, for B vitamins will keep your mind young, alert, and active.

Index

INDEX

Depression:
  biotin, 167–169
  brewer's yeast, 55
  megavitamin therapy, 165
  niacin (B-3), 171
Desiccated liver, 181, 208, 211
Diabetic skin ulcers, 85–86, 90
Diaper rash, 88, 90
Diarrhea:
  apple cider vinegar, 188
  babies and young children, 186–187
  carob powder, 187
  garlic capsules, 188
  lactobacillus acidophilus, 185, 186
  potassium gluconate, 185
  yogurt, 185, 186
Diet, recommended, 207
Digestion:
  canker sores, 188–189
    lactobacillus acidophilus, 185, 186
    yogurt, 189
  constipation, 178–182
    brewer's yeast, 178, 179, 180, 181, 182
    B vitamin complex, 180, 181, 182
    desiccated liver, 181
    foods that are born, 182
    fruits and vegetables, 182
    low-residue diet, 180
    mineral oil damaging, 179
    Three-B Program, 180–182
    unprocessed bran, 180, 181, 182
    whole wheat bread, 182
  diarrhea, 184–188
    apple cider vinegar, 188
    babies and young children, 186–187
    carob powder, 187
    garlic capsules, 188
    lactobacillus acidophilus, 185, 186
    potassium gluconate, 185
    yogurt, 185, 186
  hemorrhoids, 183–184
    vitamin E inserts, 183, 184
    vitamin E orally, 183, 184
  indigestion or heartburn, 189
    papaya tablets, 189
  raw carrot juice, 21
Doctor's Handbook of Nutritional Science,
  112

Dolomite, 48, 49, 144 (*see also* Calcium)
Drinking, 117
Dropsy, 139
Drugs, prescription, 217–218

E

E, vitamin:
  angina pectoris, 122–126
  atherosclerosis, 133
  bronchial asthma, 97
  burns, 85
  circulation in extremities, 132–133
  cramps, 144–147
  cuts, 87
  diabetic skin ulcer, 85–86, 90
  diaper rash, 88, 90
  energy, 196
  essential, 58
  fungus infection, 87, 90
  heart attack, 126–132
    after, 126–130, 131–132
    prevention, 130–131
  heart condition, 117
  hemorrhoids, 183–184
  high blood pressure, 125
  increased energy, 133
  insomnia, 151–154
  intermittent claudication, 132, 229–230
  iron neutralizes, 126
  leukoplakia, 231–232
  mineral oil dissolves, 126
  phlebitis, 132–133
  poison ivy (oak), 90
  precautions, 125–126
  rheumatic heart disease, 125–126
  scar tissue, 86, 90, 91
  shingles, 43–44
  skin, 211–213
  stay younger longer, 220, 221, 224–225
  stretch marks, 87
  sun burn, 90
  to use externally, 92
  warts, 88–89, 90
Eczema, 41–42, 90
Edema, 114–117
Eggs, 53

INDEX

INDEX

O

Older age:
    atherosclerosis, 223
    B complex vitamins, 225
    eat less, 228
    extend "prime of life," 220–221
    increase zest for life, 221–222
    intermittent claudication, 228–230
    leukoplakia, 231–232
    mental activity, 227
    mind, 232–233
    minerals, 225
    osteoporosis, 230–231
    physical activity, 227–228
    smoking, 227
    sugar, 226–227
    triglycerides, 223
    vitamins A and D, 225
    vitamin C, 220, 221, 222–224 (see also C, vitamin)
    vitamin E, 220, 221, 224–225
Osteoporosis, 230–231

P

Pain:
    insomnia, 150–151
    muscular (see Muscles)
Pain killer, 69, 118
Pancreas, 31
Pantothenic acid, 108–112
Papaya tablets, 189
Paranoia, 165, 171
Parkinson's disease, 171
Pauling, Linus, 220
Petite mal epilepsy, 169–171
Phlebitis, 132–133
Phosphorus, excess, 144
Physical activity, 227–228
Pine tar soap, scalp, 99–101
Plantar warts, 88
Pleurisy, 69
Poison ivy (oak), 90
Pollution, air, 43–44
Potassium, 201–202
Potassium chloride, 155

Potassium gluconate, 155, 185, 202
Potbelly, 214–215
Pregnancy:
    edema, B vitamins, 116
    sea kelp, 140
    wheat germ, 57
Pre-menstrual tension, 77
Prescription drugs, 217–218
Prime of life (see Older age)
Prostate gland, 30, 36–40
Psoriasis, 83–85, 90
Psychosis, 164–165
Pumpkin seeds, 38
Pyridoxine, 47–49, 118, 141–142, 170

R

Rash, 40–42, 90
Red blood cells, 107
Restless leg syndrome, 150, 152
Rheumatic heart disease, 125–126
Rheumatism:
    B vitamins, 118
    calcium, 69, 73
    cherries and cherry juice, 25
    pyridoxine (B-6), 141–142
    sea kelp, 139
Riboflavin, 171
Rose hip powder, 85
Rosenberg, Harold, 119

S

Scalp infection, 99–101
Scar tissue, 86–87, 90, 91
Schizophrenia, 165, 171
Sciatica, 171
Sea kelp, 138–140, 208
Sea salt, 155
Sedative, calcium, 69
Sex life, 215–217, 221, 222
Shingles, 42–45
Shooting pains, 144
Shute, Wilfred and Evan, 44, 56, 58
Siefert, George L., 139
Sinus congestion, 22, 31

244

INDEX

INDEX